Cancer – Your Doctor Is Not God! YOU Must Be the Battlefield General: Your 11-Step Cancer War Victory Plan

Michael Gorman

MichaelGormanBooks.com

ISBN: 9798301276545

DEDICATION

This book is dedicated to my beloved feline family, past and present: Mr. Dog, Girlie Pants, Scarlet, Miracle, Hoover, TinyCat, Squeaky, Little Bub, and Sasha.

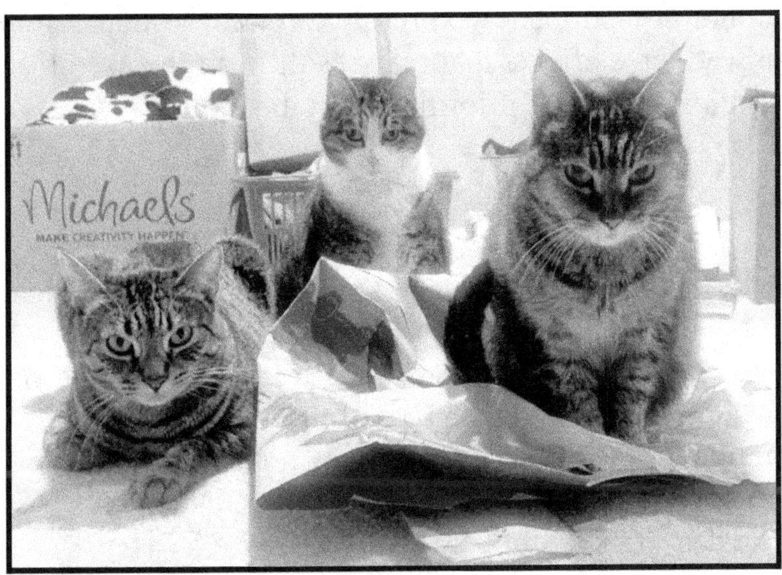

DISCLAIMER

I am not a medical professional, but a health advocate and experienced researcher. The information contained in this book is meant for informational purposes only. It is not intended to be a substitute for the advice and care of licensed medical professionals and your physician, and you should use appropriate discretion in consultation with your doctor about utilizing any of the suggestions herein as a comprehensive approach to cancer. The author and publisher expressly disclaim responsibility for any adverse effects that may result from the use or application of the information in this book.

RESEARCH FOR THIS BOOK

As a proponent of health, my personal health practices, and a health researcher, my approach is one whereby I assume there are informational errors, perhaps purposeful misinformation. To the best of my ability, I use a minimum of three corroborating and diverse sources outside myself. My goals are accuracy and truth as best as I can determine them.   MG

TABLE OF CONTENTS

PLEASE KNOW AND REMEMBER

Disclaimer

This book is a summary of my research, reviews, personal experiences, and understandings of books, videos, podcasts, and websites from physicians, oncologists, cancer research specialists, and cancer survivors.

As we begin, I want to make it clear that I am not a physician or trained healthcare specialist. This book is not to be taken as advice that supersedes that of trusted, vetted, and knowledgeable healthcare experts. As a pursuer of optimal health, active longevity, and cancer prevention, what follows are my extensive cancer research findings. Pick and choose as you will.

Suggestions here for optimizing your health and beating cancer should be thoughtfully researched and vetted by you. Groundbreaking books, podcasts, publications of health studies, cancer health websites, and the internet will aid your research, as they have mine.

To reiterate with a more legalistic precaution, the information contained in this book is meant for informational purposes only. It is not intended to be a substitute for the advice and care of licensed medical professionals and your physician, and you should use appropriate discretion in consultation with your doctor(s) about utilizing any of the suggestions herein as a comprehensive approach to cancer. The author and publisher expressly disclaim responsibility for any adverse effects that may result from the use or application of the information in this book.

MOTIVATED BY ANGER, FRUSTRATION, HOPE, AND LOVE

Why should you care about what I have to say about cancer and all that surrounds this dreaded disease --- the terrible emotional upheaval, fear, pain, treatment possibilities, depressing survival statistics, quackery, new medical technologies, and breakthrough treatments? Why should you care what I have to say? At 74, I have never faced cancer, nor has anyone in my immediate circle, family, or friends.

Why should you care about what I have to say about cancer? I am not a medical professional but a motivated and experienced researcher who views writing this book as an act of love; love for my friends and family who will go through cancer trauma, either as victims or the loving medical advocate of someone they love. This book is a loving mission to offer researched cancer treatments, curative possibilities, and cancer prevention.

My Research Background

I was a university instructor for 33 years at Oregon State University in Corvallis, and I have authored 31 books in five distinct fields, including health, history, self-betterment, cats, and fly fishing. Research is a major component of daily life.

I was given a blessed reprieve on August 3, 2022, when my 4Runner sailed off a mountain highway into a rock face, rolled over, and lay on its top in a ditch. I had fallen asleep at the wheel, literally, after three long, strenuous days of whitewater boating and fishing. I was exhausted that afternoon, and it almost cost me my life. I crawled from the mangled wreckage, sustaining only a few scratches on my left forearm.

My immediate reaction to my escape was giddiness. Those rendering medical aid and the sheriff writing his report were confused. I explained I was thrilled I had cheated death. And, it was immediately obvious to me that my life was divinely spared because I had a necessary mission: share my story and, through my writing and testimony, encourage other people to appreciate life, do and be their best, and inspire them to live optimally healthy and long, productive lives.

In 2016, I published the book *Noble Life Purpose – Discover It, Live It for a Happy Life.* I authored it under the pen name Morgan Chamile, which is discoverable at MichaelGormanBooks.com. I wrote the book for myself to discern and live my Noble Purpose, but also, of course, to help others on their journey of self-discovery and life mission fulfillment. My crash and survival again confirmed that I had important messages of inspiration, hope, and loving possibilities that needed to be shared. I view my book on cancer as part of my loving Purpose. I really have no choice and have been emphatically called to write it.

Some Recommended Authoritative & Credible Resources

I have read, and sometimes reread, scores of health and longevity books. Three of every four titles in my Audible library are about healthy living & long life. Some of my favorite health authors include Deepak Chopra, Dr. Mark Hyman, Tony Robbins, Dr. Jason Fung, G. Edward Griffin, Alexander Loyd, Dr. Marty Makary, Dave Asprey, Dr. Peter Attia, Dr. Thomas Levy, Bill Henderson, Dr. Rand McClain, Dr. Joseph Mercola, Dr. Kelly Turner, Dr. Leigh Erin Connealy, Charlotte Gerson, Mike Adams, and Ty Bollinger. ALL these experts agree that Western Medicine cancer protocols and treatments are merely a part, in many cases a small part, of your comprehensive healthcare and cancer-fighting plan.

Most recently, my reading list includes *The Truth About Cancer, Life Force, Grow Younger Live Longer, Cancer-Free, The Healing Code, Outlive, The Cancer Code: A Revolutionary New Understanding of a Medical Mystery, Dying to Be Me, World Without Cancer, How Not to Die, Super Human, Cheating Death, Food Forensics, Glucose Revolution, Blind Spots: Why We Fail to See the Solution Right in Front of Us, Healing the Gerson Way: Defeating Cancer and Other Chronic Diseases, Young Forever, Radical Remission: Surviving Cancer Against All Odds, The Cancer Revolution – A Groundbreaking Program to Reverse and Prevent Cancer,* and *The Obesity Code.* All these books have at least one significant portion dedicated to discussing and defeating cancer. I highly recommend these and other titles I will mention in this book. Many are available in audible format.

You can discover hundreds of podcasts and YouTube videos from recovering or cancer-free patients, oncologists, and researchers who offer hope and potential solutions.

Besides presenting a world of new health knowledge, treatments, therapies, and cures, all these works offer hope. Acceptance of hope and crazy-wonderful possibilities for a LONGER, active, healthy life demands a mindset change. It demands your belief in the ever-accelerating health and longevity understandings, therapies, and treatments. These are exhilarating to hear, read, and learn about.

Sadly, one common theme in EVERY health book I read is that modern Western medicine and the organizations that oversee the medical profession --- AMA, FDA, WHO, NIH --- are not paid and financed to emphasize preventative health measures and compelling, mostly inexpensive treatments; all the authors of the above-mentioned health books agree that Western medicine is about money-making. And large, wealthy pharmaceutical companies make no money when people are well. Big Pharma buys, influences, and drives medical procedures and organizations that promote their products, according to these authors, some of whom are medical doctors. Pills are about quelling symptoms more than discovering disease causes and affecting a potential reversal and cure.

All the authors and experts mentioned above often portray many medical experts, institutions, and agencies we are taught to entrust our health to as money-driven, not health-driven entities. Doctors and medical professionals can be crucial to our health but are too often limited by rules, regulations, and "governed" therapies and treatments. Again, the emphasis is that YOU must take charge of your own health.

However, this being said, if I fall and discover my broken femur protruding through my skin, I'm headed straight to a surgeon for repairs. There's no hesitation as I ponder healing alternatives. I'm on my horse or riding a lawn mower headed to the nearest hospital.

In ALL 21 health and aging books I have read in the last 2 years, the authors emphasize that individuals MUST TAKE CHARGE of their healthcare. These authors ALL believe that physicians and medical professionals play important roles but are most often focused on treating the symptoms, NOT the causes of a disease. Addressing the causes and prevention of diseases is crucial. Lifestyle changes, including diet, vitamins and supplements, physical activity, cognitive enhancement, and stress relief, are usually conspicuously absent in the standard Western medicine treatment plan. You must research, learn, and implement a comprehensive health and active longevity plan specifically tailored to you.

My Tipping Point

As I begin to write about cancer, my feelings are both mixed and passionate: frustration, sadness, anger, hope, and love. Let's start with the first three on this list.

Again, today, July 12, 2024, I listened to the continuation

of the sad story of a woman in her 50s who was suddenly diagnosed to be riddled with Stage 4 cancer in her ovaries, her liver, and her omentum, the fatty, apron-like tissue that hangs down in front of the intestines inside the abdominal cavity. A week earlier, this woman was posting photos of a vacation trip she, her husband, and their two daughters were enjoying. Now racked with pain, she is suddenly diagnosed with a spreading cancer.

With fluid quickly building inside her abdomen, today, she needs a unique medical expert with the skills to drain the fluid without doing her greater harm. Unfortunately, this fluid-draining expert is unavailable for reasons unbeknownst to my source. Sadly, a nearby hospital specializing in cancer treatment and relief has not a single bed available to help this victim, apparently unwilling to find a way to create an extra bed in the facility. Huh? How about the hallway, the spare equipment storage room, or part of the cafeteria with all those snack-dispensing vending machines? So, to relieve her of her great pain and anguish, the woman is placed into an induced coma. The husband, a man of healthy financial means, is resigned to obeying his wife's doctor and feeling helpless.

As of July 30, 2024, this woman lies in a hospital bed with a morphine drip to supposedly control her pain as she awaits more therapy. In the middle of the night, at 2 am, she texted her friend, my contact, that morphine was not quelling her physical misery, and she was unable to sleep. The patient and her family wait, then wait some more. Helpless, surrendering all treatment decisions and their timing to the doctors. She is scheduled for exploratory surgery on August 7. Why the delay as her suffering continues and her condition worsens?

When I suggested that my contact forward a potentially helpful & hope-filled cancer-specific website to the woman's fretting husband, she thought sending the website link would be an intrusion of the family's privacy and somehow out of place. My anger, which I view as righteous, and frustration are further fueled.

No less than twice in the past year, this cancer victim had sought help from her physician for abdominal pains. She was given medications for her symptoms on two occasions without an accurate assessment of the real problem, ovarian cancer, which has now spread.

As I write this sentence, it is July 31, 2024. Today, my contact referenced above has received texts from two of her friends who just had cancer surgery this week.

One woman had a cancerous melanoma cut from her scalp. During the surgery, another suspicious scalp was discovered. A sample was taken for biopsy. This begs the question: How was the newly discovered growth overlooked just weeks earlier when the confirmed cancerous mass was found? Are there other melanomas that were missed, too?

The other apparently healthy woman, friend #2, had a cancerous growth removed from her colon. She had initially sought help when rectal bleeding became evident. After the diagnosis, the woman made the decision to advocate for her health forcefully, sought additional counsel with her doctor, and *insisted* on immediate surgery. The surgeon agreed, and the job got done. This woman is a commanding general, victorious on the battlefield. Bravo!

On August 7, the woman in her early 50s with ovarian cancer mentioned above had exploratory surgery that revealed a pernicious and tragic spread of the cancer to the point where her oncologist said that more surgery would be futile in removing any of the tumors. She has been told that chemotherapy and radiation are her only options.

On August 14, I received a forwarded copy of an email from a third party written by the cancer victim's husband. "Because the cancer keeps growing aggressively, she is too weak to handle the chemotherapy, and now she can barely talk and can only open her eyes halfway. We are bedside with her to comfort her while we wait for the inevitable outcome." I interpret this as passive surrender, with no action taken.

As I continue writing here, this sad saga of passive acceptance and surrender began over a month ago. Nothing was done --- no procedures, therapies, or treatments --- in more than 30 days. The cancer was allowed to grow and spread unabated. I never heard once that the husband researched or investigated any alternative treatments that may have helped his wife. Nor did her adult daughters.

Later in this book, I reveal an expanded and comprehensive list of researched and proven IMMEDIATE / RIGHT NOW therapies, drugs, vitamins, lifestyle changes, and procedures that can be administered to the patient, most of which have no side effects with their reasonable and researched application. NONE of these possibilities require a prescription, and almost all are available at health food stores, markets, and Amazon. Not all vitamins, supplements, OTC meds, and foods are created equal. Do your research.

Here are some possible **start-immediately** treatments/therapies and three research studies supporting these cancer-fighting, noninvasive aids. As always, consider consulting trusted medical professionals.

Some Immediate/Today/Right Now Cancer-Fighting Possibilities

***Reaffirm a passionate reason, a magnificent purpose to live.** Your body, mind, and spirit ALL determine your health.

> **Bower, J. E., et al**. "Meaning in life and cancer: The role of purpose in cancer survivorship." *Psycho-Oncology,* 2021
>
> **Gonzalez, M., et al**. "The relationship between psychological resilience and cancer survival: A systematic review." *Cancer Epidemiology*, 2022
>
> **Moss, M., et al**. "Life satisfaction and its impact on cancer progression: Evidence from a longitudinal study." *Health Psychology*, 2023

***Adequate hydration with clean, purified water.** Body weight lbs. / 2 = daily fluid ounces of water

> **Lee, J. R., et al**. "Fluid intake and risk of bladder cancer." *American Journal of Epidemiology, 2008*

Wang, A. T., et al. "Fluid intake and colorectal cancer risk." *Journal of Nutrition,* 2009

Zhang, M. L. F. A., et al. "Water consumption and breast cancer risk." *Journal of Women's Health,* 2012

***Cancer-fighting and immune-enhancing, non-toxic organic foods** such as cruciferous vegetables (broccoli, cauliflower), berries, garlic, tomatoes, and green tea, to name some.

Yang, C. S., & Landau, J. M. "Tea and cancer prevention." *Nutrition and Cancer*, 2000

Porrini, M., & D'Angelo, L. "Tomatoes: A source of carotenoids and other phytochemicals with anticancer activity." Nutrients, 2015

Lin, J. K., & Lin, C. L. "The roles of garlic in the prevention of cancer." *Journal of Traditional and Complementary Medicine*, 2011

***Avoid cancer-feeding foods, such as sugar-laden foods & drinks, refined carbohydrates, and processed foods.**

Zhao, Y., et al. "Processed food consumption and cancer risk: A systematic review." *Cancer Epidemiology*, 2023

Schulze, M. B., & Hu, F. B. "Sugar-sweetened beverages and risk of cancer: A systematic review and meta-analysis." *Cancer Causes & Control*, 2020

Ma, J. et al. "Added sugar intake and cancer risk: A systematic review and meta-analysis." *Nutrition Reviews*, 2021

***Limit the use of antibiotics.**

González, J. M., et al. "Antibiotics, gut microbiota, and cancer: An emerging link." *Frontiers in Microbiology*, 2021

Sinha, R., et al. "Antibiotic use and cancer risk: A review of the evidence." *Cancer Epidemiology*, 2020.

Friedman, G. D., et al. "Antibiotic use and cancer incidence: A population-based cohort study." *Cancer Prevention Research,* 2019

***Ensure quality sleep**

Liu, Y., et al. "Sleep duration and cancer risk: A systematic review and meta-analysis." *Sleep Medicine Reviews*, 2021

Hirshkowitz, M., et al. "National Sleep Foundation's sleep time duration recommendations: Update." *Sleep Health*, 2015

Henson, J. D., et al. "Sleep quality and cancer survival: A systematic review." *Supportive Care in Cancer*, 2020

***Liposomal Vitamin C taken orally (or consider intravenous high-dose Vitamin C for patients unable to eat)**

Carr, A. C., & Frei, B. "Toward a new recommended dietary allowance for vitamin C based on antioxidant and health effects in humans." *The American Journal of Clinical Nutrition*, 1999
Chen, Q., et al. "Pharmacologic ascorbate synergizes with gemcitabine in preclinical models of pancreatic cancer." *Science Translational Medicine*, 2014
Nauman, J., et al. "Role of vitamin C in cancer treatment: A systematic review." *Nutrients*, 2020

*Vitamin D + Vitamin K

Huang, Y., et al. "Vitamin D and K2: Two Key Vitamins for Cancer Prevention." *Nutrients*, 2015
Bikle, D. D., et al. "Vitamin D: A New Player in Cancer Prevention." *Cancer Prevention Research*, 2014
Kendall, A., et al. "Vitamin D and K: Their Roles in Cancer." *Current Oncology Reports*, 2019

*B Vitamins, particularly B9 (folate)

Ducker, G. S., et al. "Emerging roles of B vitamins in cancer metabolism." *Nature*, 2016
González, C. A., et al. "B vitamins and risk of colorectal cancer: a systematic review and meta-analysis." *Cancer Causes & Control*, 2014
Kruijshaar, M. E., et al. "Folate intake and breast cancer risk: a meta-analysis." *Cancer Epidemiology, Biomarkers & Prevention*, 2012

*Quercetin

Yang, C. S., & Landau, J. M. "Quercetin and cancer prevention." *Cancer Letters*, 2000
Kumar, S., et al. "Quercetin induces apoptosis in human colon cancer cells." *Cancer Science*, 2015
Salahudeen, M. S., et al. "Quercetin inhibits cell growth and induces apoptosis in prostate cancer cells." *Biomedicine & Pharmacotherapy*, 2019

*Omega-3 Fatty Acids

Torre, L. A., et al. "Global cancer statistics, 2012." Nature Reviews Clinical Oncology, 2015
Gonzalez, M. J., & Porrini, M. "Omega-3 fatty acids and cancer." *Cancer Treatment Reviews*, 2006
Szymczak, A., et al. "Dietary Omega-3 Fatty Acids and Cancer: An Update." *Cancers*, 2019

*Turmeric/Curcumin

Hewlings, S. J., & Kalman, D. S. "Curcumin: A review of its effects on human health." *Foods*, 2017

Noble, R. E., et al. "Curcumin and its potential role in the prevention and treatment of cancer." *Cancer* Science, 2021

Goel, A., et al. "Curcumin as an anti-cancer agent: A review." *Critical Reviews in Food Science and Nutrition*, 2022

*CoQ10 (Coenzyme Q10)

Bojarczuk, C. C., et al. "Coenzyme Q10: A novel target for cancer therapy." Molecules, 2020

Rosenfeld, F. L., & Barrett, A. "Coenzyme Q10: A review of its role in cancer." *Anticancer Research*, 2021

Fuchs, M., et al. "The role of coenzyme Q10 in cancer treatment: A systematic review." *Cancers*, 2022

*NAC (N-acetylcysteine)

Wang, H., et al. "N-acetylcysteine inhibits the proliferation of cancer cells by regulating the redox status." *Biochemical and Biophysical Research Communications*, 2021

Khan, M. I., et al. "N-acetylcysteine as a potential therapeutic agent in cancer: A systematic review." *Frontiers in Pharmacology*, 2022

Torrente, L., et al. "N-acetylcysteine enhances the effects of chemotherapeutic agents in breast cancer: An in vitro study." *Journal of Cellular Physiology,* 2023

*Resveratrol

Kumar, S., et al. "Resveratrol: A potential chemo-preventive agent against cancer." *Journal of Experimental & Clinical Cancer Research*, 2021

Li, Y. et al. "Resveratrol induces apoptosis in cancer cells through the activation of the AMPK pathway." *Cancer Letters,* 2022

Gao, Y., et al. "The role of resveratrol in cancer prevention and treatment: A systematic review." *Frontiers in Pharmacology*, 2023

*Melatonin

Zhang, H., et al. "Melatonin as an anti-cancer agent: A systematic review." *Cancer Cell International*, 2021

Zhou, X., et al. "Melatonin enhances the efficacy of chemotherapy in breast cancer: An in vitro study." *Biomedicine & Pharmacotherapy*, 2022

Rovillain, E., et al. "Melatonin and its role in cancer prevention: Evidence from preclinical and clinical studies." *Cancers*, 2023

*Magnesium

Kirkland, A. E., et al. "Magnesium status and cancer: Evidence and mechanisms." *Nutrients*, 2023

Liu, Y., et al. "Magnesium intake and risk of colorectal cancer: A meta-analysis." *European Journal of Nutrition*, 2022

Zhang, H., et al. "Magnesium and cancer: A systematic review*."*
Biological Trace Element Research, 2021

Over-the-counter pain and anti-inflammatory meds like ibuprofen, naproxen, and aspirin. Research effective and reasonable doses to prevent possible side effects and optimal durations for each.

Cuzick, J., et al. "Aspirin and non-steroidal anti-inflammatory drugs (including naproxen and ibuprofen) for cancer prevention." *Cancer Prevention Research*, 2021

Rothwell, P. M., et al. "Long-term effect of aspirin on colorectal cancer incidence and mortality." *The Lancet,* 2010

Bahl, V., et al. "Aspirin and cancer: The next big thing?" *Nature Reviews Clinical Oncology*, 2013

*Stress relief techniques, including overcoming fear

Gordon, D. B., et al. "The role of stress management in cancer prevention and control: A review of the literature." *Cancer Prevention Research*, 2021

Bower, J. E., et al. "Mind-body interventions for cancer-related fatigue: A systematic review." *Psycho-Oncology*, 2022

Monti, D. A., et al. "The effects of mindfulness meditation on cancer-related outcomes: A systematic review." *Psycho-Oncology,* 2023

*Deep or power breathing

Harrison, M., et al. "The effects of deep breathing exercises on quality of life in cancer patients: A randomized controlled trial." *Journal of Cancer Research and Practice*, 2021

Carlson, L. E., et al. "The impact of a mindfulness-based intervention incorporating breathing exercises on cancer outcomes." *Psycho-Oncology*, 2023

Wang, Y., et al. "Breathing techniques and their impact on cancer-related symptoms: A systematic review." *Supportive Care in Cancer,* 2022

*Discover and remove carcinogenic environmental toxins
--- pesticides, herbicides, asbestos, radon, and toxic mold.

Gonzalez, A. J., et al. "Detection and removal of pesticides and herbicides from residential environments: A review." *Environmental Science & Technology*, 2021

Baker, E. L., et al. "Asbestos detection and management: Current practices and challenges." *Journal of Occupational and Environmental Hygiene*, 2022

Katz, S. K., et al. "Radon detection and mitigation in homes: A comprehensive approach." *Indoor Air*, 2023
***Active involvement with a caring social network and family**
Kemeny, M. E., et al. "The effects of social support on cancer outcomes: A meta-analysis." *Health Psychology*, 2019
López, J. M., et al. "Social networks, support, and cancer survival: A longitudinal study." *Cancer Epidemiology*, 2022
Kearney, J., et al. "Family involvement and quality of life in cancer patients: The role of social support." *Psycho-Oncology*, 2021
***Steam sauna therapy or steamy hot showers**
Sharma, P., et al. "Thermal therapies for cancer patients: An emerging area of interest." *Cancer Treatment Reviews*, 2022
Laukkanen, J. A., et al. "Sauna bathing and cancer incidence: A prospective cohort study." *International Journal of Cancer,* 2020
López-Quintero, C., et al. "The impact of thermal stress on immune function and cancer: A review." *Frontiers in Oncology*, 2021

Unfortunately, We Will Never Know

Would any of these have stopped the cancer's spread and helped the woman? I have no idea, but it would undoubtedly have been better, in my opinion, to try any and all of these simple, noninvasive treatments rather than take no action at all. Again, as far as I know, the husband and the woman's adult daughters did nothing to advocate for any interventions beyond what the doctor said would or wouldn't be done. Instead, the husband's note said, ". . . we wait for the inevitable outcome."

On August 17, 2024, after more than a month of little or no meaningful medical or therapeutic action to defeat the woman's cancer, she died.

I have more personal stories in which I offered friends with dying family members with cancer some cancer-specific medical resources and links to pass along. Sadly, they viewed offering such potential help as an intrusion, out of place, and possibly worthless. These friends, too, have surrendered to the idea that "the doctor knows best" because he is God. In the last year, one of the cancer victims I had hoped to help through their relative died when the man thought offering any remedy or therapy beyond what the doctor --- God --- recommended would be inappropriate, a privacy invasion.

More Sad Stories of Sickness and Cancer Death

In early 2024, at a lunch meeting with my friend Ross, he recited a long litany of his acquaintances and work colleagues who are dying or dead from cancer, most from prostate cancer. Two of my friends and fraternity brothers are dealing with prostate issues; one had a biopsy to discover if cancer was in play. Fortunately, it was not. Another longtime friend has a brother whose wife died of cancer and a brother who is fighting cancer. My neighbor's father is dying of cancer. He finally passed away on August 8. To his credit, the man, a former medical nurse, had forgone recommended radiation therapy to dedicate himself to daily walking & movement and a healthy diet. He lived for an additional 6 years.

As a longtime Boston Red Sox baseball fan, I read in a 2024 news article that former Boston pitcher Time Wakefield died a few months ago of brain cancer at age 57. Today, I read that Wakefield's wife has now died, 5 months after Tim, of pancreatic cancer.

My latest sad story, another cancer tragedy, centers around the death of a woman married to one of my high school classmates. She battled breast cancer and its fallout for several years, with my friend as her loving caregiver. Death finally took her from her suffering.

June 30, 2024, my St. Mary's Grade School class reunion. My classmate farmer friend told of his four bouts of different cancers, the latest traced to the herbicide glyphosate use. He also dealt with toxic Paraquat for decades, a poisonous, carcinogenic herbicide for killing grass and weeds.

Stories like these --- and I have many others --- make me

sad . . . frustrate me . . . make me angry. Why? Because there is tremendous hope in the form of proven treatments and approaches that cancer patients and their loved ones can't or won't consider. Because there are proven alternative possibilities, other medical cancer experts with more knowledge and treatment approaches will utilize promising breakthroughs in medical technology and cancer treatments or are willing to recommend reputable out-of-country treatment centers unfettered by American medical restrictions and prohibitions.

However, victims and their loving advocates typically fail to aggressively research, read, and listen to credible cancer researchers, most of whom are doctors, that present miraculous possibilities.

So, rise up! It's time to act with relentless purpose to discover effective help that may lead to cancer remission and even complete disappearance.

If you have not already done so, you, or one you medically advocate for, must resolve to go to war! You are not merely another soldier on the cancer battlefield. YOU are the commanding general. Physicians and medical personnel are your soldiers, your skilled and needed ground troops. Understand and embrace these respective roles.

You don't have to be a medical expert to be the commanding general. Generals don't fight the war, shoot the guns, or fly the bombers. Commanders study, they consider wise possibilities, they plan, and they give orders. If a soldier says, "Sir, we cannot win," the determined and resourceful general replies, "I have a plan, there is a way, and we WILL win!"

10 QUESTIONS FOR YOUR COMMITMENT TO WAR

The Doctor Walks In . . .

There is no more terrifying medical diagnosis on Earth.

The oncologist slowly walks through the door of the exam room to sadly announce to you, "It's cancer, and it has spread. Stage 4. At best, you have a year to live. Perhaps only months. I'm so sorry." These remarks are like a sledgehammer blow to the face. Panic and short breathing overcome you to the verge of fainting. All thoughts except one disappear from your mind: "I'm going to die, and it's probably going to be gruesome and terribly painful."

Perhaps even worse than receiving this deadly news yourself is having it delivered to someone you love — your child, your spouse, mother, father, sister, or your dearest friend.

At this pivotal life-and-death moment, you have only two immediate choices about your cancer and how to proceed: surrender or war.

If you believe the doctor is God, you can surrender to what he or she suggests as the only possible medical treatment path, hoping that prolonging your life is possible and worth the potential misery of surgery, chemotherapy, radiation, or immunotherapy. Or, perhaps, your will to live has disappeared, beaten and killed, so you surrender, choosing to do nothing.

My nonprofessional advice: CHOOSE WAR! Rather than you or your beloved dying, figuratively crying helplessly in a cold, muddy foxhole, call up your courage, summon your unbreakable will, and pick up your deadly weapons --- research, knowledge, relentless determination, planning --- and fight!

Question 1

With a cancer diagnosis, perhaps you fear that you are sentenced to a miserable, slow death with a poor quality of life in your remaining days. The question: **Do you *really* want to live, to fight the brutal war against a dirty enemy?**

Question 2

What exactly do you have to live for? That is, what will inspire you, **drive you**, to fight without wavering against an enemy that would crush your quality of life and kill you --- people whom you love and need you, a mission, a cause, or important unfinished goals?

Question 3

If you do not believe you can beat cancer, your belief can be your doom. "As you think, so you are." Motivation and action begin in the mind and are fueled by hope and belief. Growing and solidifying your hope is an excellent first step toward creating your Master Health Plan.

There is an avalanche of new medical technologies, innovative cancer therapies, promising new drugs, and a growing research-based understanding of what cancer is and how to reverse the disease. Countless victorious testimonies from cancer survivors are found in books, podcasts, websites, and YouTube.

I recently finished the book *Dying to Be Me* by Anita Moorjani. In it, she tells her story of terminal cancer that completely decimated her body. Comatose in her last hours, she tells of her near-death experience and the choice she made to return to her earthly life. In a few days --- proven with unassailable medical records and medical staff testimonies --- the cancer completely disappeared. She testifies to overcoming impossibilities.

Moorjani attributes her recovery to a profound spiritual

awakening during a near-death experience. She emphasizes that her healing was linked to embracing self-love, authenticity, and letting go of fear. She believes that by accepting herself and releasing her emotional burdens, she created an environment conducive to healing. Her journey illustrates the power of mindset, belief, and emotional well-being in the face of illness.

These sources and stories are all easily discovered if you take the time to find them. Hope abounds!

Now, the question you must answer: **Do you believe deeply that you can beat your cancer?**

Question 4

A lukewarm determination will not suffice against a merciless enemy. **Do you have the tenacious will and commitment to fight, study, plan, and execute a war to save your life or the life of your loved one?**

Question 5

A successful Battle Plan will demand extensive research, investigating many different credible sources, reading, listening to, or watching cancer survivor success stories, searching websites dedicated to cancer-beating strategies and therapies, formulating an effective Battle Plan, and giving the orders necessary to carry out a successful war. **Are you committed to do the work?**

Question 6

Cancer has many causes, 90% of which --- according to credible experts cited here, among many other cancer researchers --- are related to diet, obesity, physical inactivity, stress, and environmental toxins. 90%!!!!!! Understanding your cancer's cause is imperative to its defeat and the prevention of its recurrence. **As part of your healing and restoration journey, are you open to courageously**

exploring the possibility that YOU caused or allowed your cancer?

Question 7

Medical errors, botched surgeries, misdiagnoses, or prescribing incorrect or deadly drugs or therapies are the *third leading cause of death* in the United States! 250,000 Americans die every year from doctor-related errors. (More details later in this book) Just because your doctor pronounces that your Earthly time is limited or that you have only one or two cancer therapeutic choices does NOT necessarily make it true. **Are you willing to acknowledge that your doctor is not God?** Your life may depend on it.

Question 8

No one cares as much about your recovery and defeat of your cancer as you or your loving advocate. So, YOU, or your advocate, must be the commanding battlefield general in the cancer war. You, the General, or your advocate general, will study, plan, prosecute the war and make necessary adjustments as needed. **Are you determined to take control of your health and be the informed decision-maker, the commanding general, on how to defeat your cancer?**

Note: Your doctor(s) is a necessary soldier in this war. Consider their knowledge, experience, and recommendations, but you must ultimately decide for yourself to agree to or consider other credible medical opinions and alternative healing therapies. Again, your life depends on it.

Question 9

The motivational tipping point that drove me to write this book was the story of a woman in her 50s who twice pleaded for a thorough examination of her abdominal pain. She was given painkillers to treat her symptoms, but no diagnosis was determined. Her mishandled complaints may ultimately lead to her death, as I write this sentence in August 2024. Once her ovarian cancer had been discovered months after her original complaints, she lay in her hospital bed waiting, waiting, waiting in intense pain for weeks for her next procedure, an exploratory surgery. It was revealed on August 7 that the cancer had spread and worsened in the weeks she lay there and suffered. Neither the woman nor her husband insisted on immediate action, a second opinion, or immediate or alternative treatment at another medical facility. More on her story later.

So, as the Commanding General in your cancer war, or on behalf of someone you love, after the necessary research and consideration of credible healing sources . . . **Are you willing to demand immediate action NOW, find another doctor, travel to another treatment center, or demand alternative therapies and treatments NOW, not next month?**

Question 10

I have heard from too many ill people unwilling to pay for expensive travel, relocation, and treatments. They often have the money but are reluctant to spend it saving their own life. We have all heard the adage, "You can't take it with you." **Are you willing to dedicate the financial resources required to save your life?**

Let's Start Planning the War Now, General!

The following pages will help you understand your enemy, prepare you to confront the inevitable obstacles, create and execute a successful battle plan against your cancer, and offer you hope and encouragement to win this war.

YOUR DOCTOR IS NOT GOD!

You must refuse to be ordinary, refuse to be normal, and go against what the vast majority of Earthlings believe: oncologists, doctors, and the "knowledgeable and learned" medical experts are gods. You may think these gods went through years of medical school and learned all that exists about skillfully treating disease. They did not.

Interestingly, the vast majority of physician authors and podcasters I've read and listened to agree that traditionally trained Western doctors are bound by institutional constraints and limitations. They contend that Western medicine is limited and hamstrung by regulations and laws that disable them from considering possible effective therapies, treatments, drugs, and nutrition that can affect cancer remission, healing, and even cures. More on these later.

Ignoring the Obvious

Dr. Marty Makary, Johns Hopkins Surgeon and author of the bestseller *Blind Spots:* "I didn't spend a second in medical school talking about nutrition. It wasn't taught."

The typical duration of U.S. medical school education is four years. This is usually divided into two phases: pre-clinical and clinical, as well as hands-on educational experience. In addition to my personal inquiries with medical professionals, here are three sources that indicate the insanely brief teaching of the health importance of nutrition in a **4-year** medical education:

***Srinivasan, M., et al**. (2013) - Their study published in Medical Education found that most U.S. medical schools dedicate an average of **19.6 hours** to nutrition education over the entire curriculum, highlighting the need for increased emphasis on nutrition in medical training.

***Rochon, J., et al**. (2016) - This study published in *The Journal of Nutrition* indicated that the time allocated to nutrition education in U.S. medical schools averaged about **24 hours**, but the content and delivery varied significantly between institutions.

***Schilling, L., et al**. (2017) - Research in *BMC Medical Education* reported that the average time spent on nutrition education across 15 medical schools was approximately **23 hours**, emphasizing the inconsistency in training and the call for improvement.

As a provocative hypothetical, I am supposing a medical student, in their average 4-year schooling, is in the classroom or medical facility 6 hours/day, 30 hours/week, 50 weeks/year for 4 years. 30 hours/week x 50 weeks x 4 years = 6,000 hours of medical education. Compare a pitiful 24-hour average maximum of nutrition education to 6,000 hours of total medical education!!!!

Expressed another way, for every 250 hours of medical education, 1 hour was dedicated to healthy, immunity-enhancing, disease-preventing nutrition.

Seeking additional related information, I researched the average number of nutrition education hours for those seeking a *naturopathic* medical degree.

Here are my sources:

***Agboola, P. A. L., Alwan, S. M., & McMillan, M. A.** (2016). "Nutrition education in naturopathic medical education: A review of accredited programs." *Journal of Naturopathic Medicine*: 100 – 200 hours.

***Doe, K. A., & Smith, J. C.** (2018). "Naturopathic nutrition education: Curriculum analysis and implications." *Journal of Naturopathic Medicine*: 90 – 120 hours.

***Sullivan, M. A. D. L. M., & Haverly, K. R. H.** (2017). "Training in holistic medicine: A survey of nutrition education." *American Journal of Lifestyle Medicine*: 50 – 150 hours.

Taking the average of the three hourly ranges in the research studies above would indicate a possible average of 118 hours of nutrition education for naturopath doctors compared to the average of 24 hours for mainstream "standard" physicians. This would translate to almost 500% more nutrition education time by the naturopaths. This is one more important reason to have a naturopathic physician as one of the medical soldiers on your team.

Why the Focus on Food?

Why have I singled out nutrition as an essential cancer-related educational topic? Because EVERY source, author, researcher, and website referenced in this book cites healthy nutrition & diet as critical to fighting and preventing cancer. I contend that what I, a nonmedical layman, have learned --- and continue to learn --- about a healthy diet has easily spanned many hundreds of hours. So, I have a question: When was the last time --- if ever --- your physician consulted with you about changing your diet to head off or cure your disease or ailment, including cancer?

This then begs a follow-up question: How many other relevant prevention and curative treatments, specifically related to cancer, are not adequately addressed in medical schools?

Do You Still Believe? Don't!

Still want to believe doctors are God? Let me present you with a telling and authoritative research study supporting my case that doctors are not gods. I am presenting a statistic here that I researched and wrote about in one of my previous books, *I Said "Hell No!" to the Grim Reaper – 200 Health Hacks for Your Optimal Health and Living Robustly Beyond 100 Years.* (Available at MichaelGormanBooks.com)

A 2016 study by researchers at Johns Hopkins University estimated that more than 250,000 people in the US die every year due to medical errors, including surgical, medication, anesthesia, and misdiagnosis events. The research was led by Dr. Martin Makary, a professor of surgery at the Johns Hopkins University School of Medicine. The researchers examined four studies that analyzed medical death rate data from 2000 to 2008 and extrapolated their findings using hospital admission rates from 2013. The researchers point out that the Centers for Disease Control and Prevention's (CDC) method of collecting national health statistics fails to classify medical errors separately on death certificates. The 250,000 death figure ranks medical errors as the **third leading cause of death** in the United States, behind heart disease and cancer and ahead of respiratory disease. According to their calculations, medical errors accounted for 9.5 percent of all deaths each year in the US, almost 1 in 10.

As a pertinent side note on nutrition ignorance or carelessness, the Johns Hopkins research leader, Dr. Marty Makary, in his book *Blind Spots: When Medicine Gets it Wrong, and What it Means for Our Health*, references food commonly provided to ill patients in a hospital where he worked: "I was perplexed by how we responded to hungry patients who begged us for food. We'd feed them small portions of Jello and flavorless processed food, a human rights violation by some definitions."

In a November 2024 video interview on Rumble.com entitled "America's Food Is Poison", with Dr. Makary, the interviewer asks the Johns Hopkins surgeon, "Can we trust the 'medical establishment' in America anymore?"

Makary: "Public trust in doctors and hospitals is way down according to a survey that was just done a month ago. It's down from 71% (in 2020) to 40% (in 2024)." The survey (with more than 582,000 responses, published in JAMA Open Network July 2024) was "a little peek that the public got on to how a broader "medical priesthood" works." Makary goes on, "When it comes to health, we have conditioned doctors to really just use medications and a scalpel."

Hmmm. Johns Hopkins University School of Medicine, where Makary works and does research. Is this institution and its medical staff reputable?

To address this issue, I proposed the following query for an internet search, including various artificial intelligence chatbots: "List the top 10 most prestigious medical schools in the US." Every listing I viewed had Johns Hopkins in Baltimore, Maryland ranked at #2 or #3. For perspective, there are no less than 195 accredited U.S. medical schools.

My point here is that doctors and medical practitioners are not all-knowing and infallible if, on average, a quarter of a million Americans die annually as a result of medical errors, including surgical, medication, anesthesia, and misdiagnosis of ailments and diseases.

This crazy stat is provided here to push YOU into being your primary medical advocate, rather than merely relying on a physician, including a cancer specialist, who says surgery, chemotherapy, and radiation are your only options for your cancer treatment or the cancer treatment of your beloved. Or, worse yet, the oncologist says, "You have months to live, so get your affairs in order and say goodbye to your family and friends," and you assume the battle is lost and the war is over. Because "the doctor says so" doesn't make it necessarily true.

Remember, a quarter of a million Americans die each year from medical errors, and perhaps your doctor is in error. Your doctor isn't God. Your life, or that of your charge, is at stake. Take charge. After an initial diagnosis and treatment recommendations, start by getting two, three, or four more opinions as you fashion your battle plan.

Along with the theme emphasized in the title of this book, Dr. Marty Makary in *Blind Spots* emphasizes the importance of patient empowerment by stating that patients should be active participants in their healthcare decisions, advocating for informed choices, and open communication with their healthcare providers. He encourages individuals to take charge of their health and to ask questions about their treatment options.

Furthermore, Makary recommends that cancer treatment should involve **a team** of specialists from various fields to create comprehensive treatment plans tailored to the individual's specific situation. Certainly, I concur when a cancer diagnosis is received. One opinion and treatment perspective are never sufficient. Recruit as many valuable soldiers as possible to fight in your war.

A Grade School Memory

I remember a grade school kid a few years older than me who was anesthetized while a surgeon worked on his broken arm. George never woke up. He died on the operating table to repair a broken bone. Was it a medical error? Maybe. Maybe not. That was never determined.

You have an important and necessary say in your medical treatment. Be thoughtful, researched, and respectfully assertive. Refuse to be an ordinary and obediently compliant sheep. Yes, medical experts and doctors can add to your health and even save your life, but they are only part of your health Master Plan.

Another Tragic Medical Anecdote

In 2024, I was told the story of a teeneager who was injured in a family logging accident. The tip of a broken tree limb became embedded in his shoulder. Taken immediately to a hospital, a surgeon removed the wood and closed the wound. The boy remained in the hospital and quickly developed a serious fever, demanding further cleaning of the wound.

With the fever persisting, the concerned parents wanted their son transported to a larger medical facility with more resources where other doctors with perhaps a different view of the boy's deterioration might successfully treat him. Their pleedings were denied and the parents relented.

Unfortunately, within five days of his initial treatment and continuous stay in the hospital, the teeneager died. I cannot begin to imagine the possible regret and immortal anguish now lived by the parents who acquiesced to the boy's surgeon and the hospital, which ultimately led to his death.

A Small Take-Charge Example

At the time of my 2023 annual physical exam, I related to my physician that I had a couple of issues with my left ear.

For almost a year, I had a persistent itch at the entrance to my ear canal, and my left ear was plugged, with my hearing muffled like when swimmers sometimes retain water in their ears. So, I was prescribed an antifungal medication that would hopefully remedy both problems. It didn't.

Next step: I was referred to an ENT (Ear Nose & Throat) specialist. I waited for the ENT office to call to schedule an appointment as I was told they would. In the meantime, I continued to experiment with a variety of over-the-counter ear drops and nasal inhalants. Nothing worked. My left ear itched and my hearing in that ear was still muffled.

On a whim --- please remember I am not a doctor or a medical pro, so know this is NOT medical advice --- I put a few drops of a colloidal silver *nasal* spray barely inside my ear canal. The experiment soon cured the persistent itching. Hmmm.

After weeks of waiting for a call that never came from the ENT office, I kept researching the internet and YouTube about plugged ear remedies. I then took it upon myself to buy a $39 over-the-counter commonly available device for gently injecting air into my nostrils. After my **first** use of the tool, which was intended to equalize the pressure in my nasal passage, my hearing miraculously returned.

Do these personal anecdotes mean disregarding professional medical help? No. Be assured that I will not be my first choice to extract a bullet from my abdomen and dress the wound or re-attach an ear severed in a landscaping project.

THE CANCER RESEARCH & PRACTIONER ALL-STAR TEAM

Dr. Marty Makary

Dr. Marty Makary is a prominent surgeon, author, and healthcare expert affiliated with Johns Hopkins University. Makary earned his M.D. from Wake Forest University School of Medicine and a master's degree from Harvard University. He completed his residency at Johns Hopkins Hospital.

Makary is a fellow of the American College of Surgeons. His research focuses on patient safety, healthcare quality, and the impact of transparency in healthcare, including his research referenced earlier showing that medical errors and malpractice stands as the third-leading cause of American deaths, and has been involved in initiatives aimed at reducing medical errors and improving the quality of care in hospitals.

He has authored books including *Unaccountable: What Hospitals Won't Tell You and How Transparency Can Revolutionize Health Care* (2012) in which he discusses the lack of transparency in the healthcare system and advocates for reforms to improve patient safety and care. In his *The Price We Pay: What Broke American Health Care and How to Fix It* (2019) he examines the healthcare system's flaws and offers solutions for reform, focusing on cost, accessibility, and quality of care. Finally, in *Blind Spots: Why We Fail to See the Solution Right in Front of Us* (2021) he writes of the reasons behind systemic failures in healthcare and emphasizes the importance of accountability and innovative solutions.

In November 2024, Makary was nominated to head the Food and Drug Administration (FDA).

Dr. Thomas Seyfried

Seyfried received his PhD in Genetics and Biochemistry from the University of Illinois Urbana-Champaign in 1976. He completed a postdoctoral fellowship and served as an assistant professor in neurology at Yale University School of Medicine. Now, I am a professor of biology at Boston College. He has a broad presence on YouTube and popular podcast platforms. Seyfried has conducted scores of informative published interviews, many of which I have watched or listened to.

Research focus and writings: Seyfried's work centers on mechanisms of chronic diseases, particularly cancer, epilepsy, neurodegenerative lipid storage diseases, and caloric restriction diets. He wrote *Cancer as a Metabolic Disease: On the Origin, Management, and Prevention of Cancer,* published in 2012. Dr. Seyfried has authored over 150 peer-reviewed publications. He leads a lab at Boston College focusing on dietary therapies for epilepsy, cancer, and neurodegenerative lipid storage diseases.

Note of interest: In late November 2024, Dr. Marty Makary was nominated by President-elect Donald Trump to be the head of the US Food and Drug Administration (FDA).

Dr. Jason Fung

A Canadian, Fung received his medical degree from the University of Toronto and completed his residency in internal medicine and a fellowship in nephrology. He's worked in various medical settings, including hospitals and clinics, focusing on treating kidney disease, obesity, and cancer.

Research focus and writings: As the author of the books *The Cancer Code: A Revolutionary New Understanding of a Medical Mystery* and *The Obesity Code,* Fung's insights into cancer and metabolic health draw on both his clinical experience and research in these areas.

Dr. Mark Hyman

Hyman received his Doctor of Medicine (MD) degree from the University of Ottawa, Faculty of Medicine in Canada. He is the head of Strategy and Innovation at the Cleveland Clinic Center for Functional Medicine and the founder and director of The UltraWellness Center, a functional medicine practice in Massachusetts.

He has written several best-selling books on health and wellness, including *The Blood Sugar Solution 10-Day Detox Diet, Eat Fat, Get Thin, The UltraMind Solution,* and *Food: What the Heck Should I Eat?*

Besides being frequently interviewed on YouTube and other platforms, Hyman is a podcaster and host of *The Doctor's Farmacy*. I highly recommend it.

Dr. Thomas Levy, MD

Author of the book *Curing the Uncurable*: *Vitamin C, Infectious Disease, and Toxins*, Levy earned his MD from Tulane University School of Medicine and is a board-certified cardiologist. He also holds a law degree (JD) from Tulane University Law School.
Levy has focused much of his research and writing on the therapeutic uses of high-dose vitamin C, advocating for its use in treating infections, chronic diseases, and toxin exposure. In addition to *Curing the Incurable*, he has authored several other books and lectures internationally on vitamin C and health.

Dr. Kelly Turner

Dr. Turner holds a B.A. from Harvard University and a Ph.D. from the University of California, Berkeley. Her doctoral research focused on the phenomenon of spontaneous remission of cancer, where she conducted interviews with healers, doctors, and cancer survivors across ten countries.

Her best-selling *Radical Remission: Surviving Cancer*

Against All Odds is a book in which Turner explores the stories and common factors among individuals who have experienced unexpected remission from cancer. Based on Turner's research and interviews with over a thousand cancer patients, the book identifies 10 key factors that these survivors often share.

Turner created, co-produced, and directed *Radical Remission*, a 10-part docuseries that explores the ten healing factors from her research and features many Radical Remission survivors from her books. The series is streaming exclusively on HayHouse.com.

Turner is the founder of the Radical Remission Project, a website and online community that continues to collect new cases of Radical Remission and offers online courses, in-person workshops, and one-on-one health coaching by 150+ certified Radical Remission health coaches from around the world.

Dr. Peter Attia

Dr. Peter Attia earned his Doctor of Medicine (M.D.) degree from Stanford University School of Medicine. He completed his residency in General Surgery at Johns Hopkins Hospital and spent two years as a Surgical Oncology Fellow at the National Cancer Institute (NCI), part of the National Institutes of Health (NIH).

Attia co-authored *Outlive: The Science and Art of Longevity* (2023). This book covers various aspects of longevity, including how lifestyle, diet, exercise, and advanced medical interventions can extend lifespan and improve quality of life. While not exclusively about cancer and its prevention and treatment, he certainly addresses cancer prevention and management at length. He is frequently featured on popular health podcasts and YouTube.

Dr. Leigh Erin Connealy

The author of *The Cancer Revolution – A Groundbreaking Program to Reverse and Prevent Cancer*, Leigh Connealy, earned her Medical Doctor (MD) degree from the University of Texas Medical Branch in Galveston and has pursued additional training in Integrative and Functional Medicine, which focuses on combining conventional medical approaches with alternative therapies to treat the whole person, considering lifestyle, nutrition, and environmental factors.

Connealy has specialized training in advanced cancer therapies and integrative oncology, emphasizing her expertise in using both traditional and alternative methods to address cancer.

Charlotte Gerson

Gerson is a proponent and educator of the Gerson Therapy, which is based on the research, treatments, and protocols pioneered and laid out by her father, Dr. Max Gerson (1881-1959), a German physician who dedicated his life to understanding cancer and developing therapies he showed effective in its treatment. His primary research and work took place in the 1940s and 50s.

Charlotte is the founder of the Gerson Institute, an organization that promotes the Gerson Therapy worldwide, and an author and lecturer on natural healing, detoxification, and cancer treatments. She wrote *Healing the Gerson Way: Defeating Cancer and Other Chronic Diseases*, first published in 2005. This book is a guide to the Gerson Therapy, a natural, holistic treatment focusing on nutrition, detoxification, and lifestyle changes to treat chronic diseases, particularly cancer. The book offers practical instructions on implementing the Gerson Therapy, including diet recommendations, juicing, and detox methods like coffee enemas.

Ty Bollinger

After the cancer deaths of his father, both grandfathers, and four other family members, researcher, and author Ty Bollinger dedicated "thousands of hours" (his words) to learning all he could about cancer, its cause, the bodily environment that encourages its growth, alternative treatment clinics including out-of-country facilities, and the discovery of effective diet and lifestyle protocols to attack it and defeat cancer. As a result, he wrote his informative and popular book, *The Truth About Cancer.*

Bollinger says, "I lost my entire family to cancer. I don't believe I had to lose them." He states that *The Truth About Cancer* has been written for one simple reason: to share the knowledge we need to protect ourselves, treat ourselves, and, in some cases, save our lives or the lives of those we love. His October 2015 documentary miniseries *The Truth About Cancer: A Global Quest* has received over 5 million views. It explains that there are many methods we can access to treat and prevent cancer that are yet to be discovered.

Key themes of Bollinger's book and his docuseries include:
*The history and politics of cancer treatment.
*A myriad of natural and alternative cancer therapies.
*Personal stories and testimonies from cancer survivors.
*Criticisms of the pharmaceutical industry and mainstream medical practices.

Dr. Joseph Mercola

Dr. Mercola earned his Doctor of Osteopathy (D.O.) degree from the Chicago College of Osteopathic Medicine at Midwestern University. He is licensed as an osteopathic physician, focusing on holistic and preventative care.

He has authored several health, nutrition, and wellness books, many of which have become bestsellers. He wrote *Fat for Fuel: A Revolutionary Diet to Combat Cancer, Boost*

Brain Power, and Increase Your Energy" (2017), in which Mercola advocates for a ketogenic diet, intermittent fasting, and maintaining the healthy function of the cell's mitochondria, their energy-producing organelles.

In his *Effortless Healing,* Mercola further discusses various health strategies, including dietary changes, that he claims can help prevent and treat cancer.

A third book of interest is Mercola's *Emotional Freedom Technique (EFT) for Cancer* (2010). This book focuses on using EFT, a form of psychological acupressure, to reduce stress and emotional trauma, which he believes can contribute to cancer development and hinder healing. He emphasizes the importance of mental and emotional health in cancer prevention and treatment.

He founded Mercola.com, a website that promotes various health and wellness strategies, emphasizing alternative and natural treatments.

Dr. Tom Rogers

Oncologist Dr. Tom Rogers received his medical degree at the University of Toronto. He has participated in specialized training and fellowships related to cancer treatment and research, further enhancing his expertise in the field.

In addition to his clinical work, he is involved with and contributes to studies that advance the understanding of cancer biology and treatment options. Rogers' YouTube channel combines his medical background with a passion for educating the public about cancer and related health issues, emphasizing evidence-based information.

CancerChoices.org

CancerChoices.org is a tremendous cancer patient resource dedicated to providing care and support for individuals affected by this disease. It offers comprehensive information on various treatment options, including conventional and integrative therapies. The platform emphasizes holistic approaches to healing, considering physical, emotional, and spiritual well-being in its numerous articles, experts' insights, personal stories, and practical guidance. The overriding goal of the site is to empower individuals with knowledge and hope, encouraging informed decisions and enhancing the overall quality of life during and after treatment.

11-STEP CANCER-FIGHTING MASTER BATTLE PLAN

Step 1: A Warrior's Mindset

Tenacious Commitment to Living

Physical pain, emotional pain, fear, and clinical depression can be overwhelming. One or all of these can incapacitate a person to the point they cannot think clearly and take focused action on a plan that might end their suffering and move them toward healing. The cancer patient can be consumed with mental and physical misery to exclude anything else. Add fear to these, and you have a toxic mix that leads to surrender, a resignation to suffering, and perhaps death. Sadly, many cancer sufferers welcome death as their only relief.

The immediate challenge in taking charge of your health and healing demands successfully overcoming your pain and fear. How can this be done from an emotional and pain-filled cesspool? Pain-killing drugs may be part of the answer, but they can also be a significant detriment to awareness, clear thinking, and necessary war-winning determination.

The Loving Patient Advocate

If you are reading this book from the viewpoint of a loving advocate interceding on behalf of a cancer victim unable to fight for themselves, then YOU are the battlefield commander. What I am suggesting to successfully prosecute the war is now in your hands. Love is your noble motivation. Refuse anything less than complete victory, General.

A Committed Warrior

Beating cancer, optimizing your health, and working towards living actively and happily must be driven by powerful reasons to do the work, summon the discipline, create a sound health plan, and overcome the many challenges that must overcome on your journey. You must have a valiant warrior's mindset. Banish laziness and shortcuts. Don't accept merely one opinion about healing and wellness. Never!

What is your powerful incentive, your motivation? What will drive You toward victory for optimal health and winning the cancer war? You must have at least one passionate reason. If you have an unhappy and/or unfulfilling life, why would you want work to extend it? You won't.

Answer some questions: Who needs you? Who wants you to live because they love you and you love them? What thrills you? What or who makes you happy and gives you joy that motivates you to live? What must you see, visit, experience, and do before you can ever leave this Earth? What knowledge, skills, and gifts do you have that the World wants and needs?

Driven by Your Noble Purpose

You have a Noble Purpose, a calling to give yourself, your talents, and your love to the world. If you have not, discover, define, and live it. See living as an act of love, love of the world and yourself. Defining and living your Noble Purpose can drive you to pursue healing, optimal health, and a long life because you are on a sacred mission.

As just mentioned, in 2016, I published the book *Noble Life Purpose – Discover It, Live It for a Happy Life*, motivated primarily to discover and live my Noble Purpose and help others on their journey of self-discovery and life mission fulfillment. Part of my Noble Purpose is writing this book to help you discover *your* Noble Purpose.

You may say, "What do I really have to offer? I have few desirable skills or talents anyone needs or cares about." To this, I would tell you that you have much to offer the world, especially as one who challenged and held cancer in check, fought for life, and won. How inspirational is that! People respond to the victory and hope you relate. And living your Noble Purpose can involve expressions as simple as smiling with direct eye contact at all you encounter passing on the sidewalk or strolling the isles of Walmart. Everyone responds to your smile. It lifts their spirit, endorphins flow, and the immune system is boosted. Of course, you may also want to write an inspirational book, make uplifting YouTube videos, or go on a nationwide speaking tour to tell your story. There are no limits!

But you may say, "I don't want to live in a painful, feeble state. The same is true for my sick family member or good friend. There will be no quality of life." My response to you, then, is there are countless stories of people who beat cancer and recovered to live and enjoy an active, pain-free life. Check out YouTube. There are many, many encouraging testimonials from cancer survivors who fought the cancer war and won. Most had to work diligently to overcome challenges and obstacles, including themselves. There is great hope.

Be a motivated, will-not-be-denied warrior. Do your research, create a Master Plan, and execute it. Hope and healing are yours. Make yourself and those you advocate for proud of you.

Believe that Healing and Cancer Abatement Are Possible, Even Likely

If you do not believe you can beat cancer, your belief can be your doom. "As you think, so you are." Motivation and action begin in the mind and are fueled by hope and belief. Growing and solidifying your hope is an excellent first step toward creating your Master Health Plan.

A simple passive way to begin believing you can thwart cancer is to view an endless number of cancer survivor testimonials available on YouTube. Merely search "cancer survivor," "how I beat cancer." or "I beat cancer." Hear from the mouths of those warriors who fought the cancer war and won. These are guaranteed to lift your spirit, give you hope, and summon your willpower. Additionally, you will notice recurrent themes of the healing process, such as dietary changes, movement & exercise, emotional positivity, hydration, stress relief, and quality sleep, among others. These are all lifestyle facets over which YOU have control, even in a hospital bed.

Cancer researcher Dr. Kelly Turner, whom you will read more about in the coming pages, specializes in integrative oncology and has extensively researched cases of radical cancer remission, which occurs when cancer patients recover in statistically unlikely ways without conventional medicine or after conventional treatments have failed. Over the past decade, she has analyzed more than 1,500 cases of radical remission. She summarized her findings in her York Times bestselling book *Radical Remission: Surviving Cancer Against All Odds*, available in 23 languages. She created a list of 10 cancer healing protocols, which she discovered to be shared by most of the survivors she interviewed. None of the 10 include chemotherapy or radiation, though these too may be part of your healing Master Plan.

I will address proven lifestyle and nutritional recommendations from Turner and other brilliant cancer researchers in the following pages and again in summary at this book's conclusion.

The Healing Power of Belief

Simply believing that healing from cancer is a possibility will aid your body in fighting your cancer. I have just referenced a few sources of cancer survivor testimonials. They are proof that beating cancer is doable.

The concept of the "power of belief" as it relates to cancer often intersects with fields like psychoneuroimmunology and mind-body medicine. Research in these areas explores how psychological factors, such as beliefs and attitudes, can influence cancer outcomes. Here are three notable scientific research examples that illustrate the impact of belief and psychological factors on cancer:

The Placebo Effect and Cancer Treatment

A landmark study published in the Journal of Clinical Oncology (2010) explored the placebo effect in cancer treatment. The study, "Placebo Effect and the Effect of the 'Nocebo' Effect in Clinical Trials of Anticancer Agents," examined how patients' expectations and beliefs could affect their response to treatment. The research found that patients who believed they were receiving effective treatment often experienced improved outcomes, even when they were actually receiving a placebo. This effect is attributed to the brain's ability to influence physiological processes through expectation and belief. The study underscores how the placebo effect can significantly impact patients' experiences and potentially their responses to actual treatments.

Mindfulness-Based Stress Reduction (MBSR) and Cancer

A study published in the Journal of Clinical Oncology (2004), titled "Mindfulness-Based Stress Reduction for the Prevention of Depression, Anxiety, and Stress in Cancer Survivors," investigated the effects of mindfulness practices on cancer patients. The study demonstrated that MBSR, which involves techniques such as meditation and mindfulness, could help reduce symptoms of anxiety, depression, and stress in cancer patients. Participants who engaged in MBSR reported improved quality of life and better emotional regulation. The research suggests that mindfulness and the belief in its benefits can positively influence patients' overall well-being and potentially improve cancer treatment outcomes.

Optimism and Cancer Survival

A study published in the Cancer Research Journal (2007), titled "Optimism and Survival in Patients with Breast Cancer," examined the impact of optimism on survival rates in breast cancer patients. The study found that breast cancer patients with a higher level of optimism had significantly better survival rates than those with lower optimism levels. The research suggests that positive psychological factors, including belief in recovery and a hopeful outlook, can influence cancer progression and survival. The mechanisms are thought to involve immune system functioning and stress response, both of which are influenced by psychological states.

Conclusion About Healing & Hope

These studies provide evidence that psychological factors, such as belief, expectation, and optimism, can have a tangible impact on cancer outcomes. While belief alone is not a substitute for medical treatment, it can complement therapies by improving emotional well-being, reducing stress, and potentially influencing physiological responses. These boost the immune system's ability to fight cancer. This highlights the importance of integrating psychological support into cancer care.

Here's a truism that naturally follows: "If you believe you can, you are correct. If you believe you can't, you are correct." Applying this quip to the disease, if you believe your doctor is God and you *believe* him when he says you are going to die, you are likely correct. If you *believe* there is a curative answer to your cancer, you are probably correct.

Step 2 --- Anticipate and Plan for Roadblocks and Challenges

The Necessity of Assertiveness

To stand up confidently for yourself and your health against the opinions and advice of your doctor and other medical professionals starts with knowledge. Listen to testimonials of cancer survivors on YouTube, read books like those I have referenced, watch or listen to the countless interviews of researchers and cancer experts while you discover recurrent healing and cancer-eradication themes. When your doctor says that surgery, chemotherapy, and radiation are your only options, you will be ready. If 95% of survivors and cancer researchers say that changing your diet is crucial to healing and recovery, but your doctor has made no mention of diet or the importance of being adequately hydrated, this should give you pause. How can any cancer physician overlook obvious simple cancer-fighting protocols?

Instead of being passively obedient, ask questions and relate to the oncologist what you heard from cancer survivors who opted out of traditional Western treatments and lived or are living well beyond their predicted survival years. Ask about the health-harming side effects of chemotherapy and radiation, both of which weaken our first line of defense against cancer, the immune system. What about immunotherapy, hyperbaric oxygen therapy, or fasting? You have a right to know the answers to all your questions.

Always insist on a second opinion. Remember, a quarter of one million Americans die each year due to medical errors, including prescribing the wrong treatments for potentially fatal diseases.

Knowledge about cancer and a myriad of protocols to defeat it are magnificent fuels for your assertiveness. Read, listen, watch, and learn. Then, demand, if necessary.

Challenges from Our Human Nature

You MUST mentally prepare for roadblocks and challenges on the battlefield that will assuredly come. Change your perspective. View challenges as opportunities.

Inertia is a term from physics. It is resistance to motion, to movement. Sir Isaac Newton --- the apple-fell-on-my-head guy and cat lover --- put together some physics-related tenants. Newton's First Law of Motion states that an object at rest (you and me) tends to stay at rest until acted on by a force (like a motivating thought).

Laziness is the perfect human example of inertia. Author and psychiatrist M. Scott Peck wrote a self-help book that sold 10 million copies. Released in 1978, *The Road Less Traveled*, which I have read four times, relates the challenges Peck and his psychotherapy patients commonly encountered as they worked together toward restoring the client, as best as possible, to a mentally and emotionally full, functional life. Peck offers the reader his insights, advice, and philosophy toward creating a better life.

In *The Road Less Traveled*, Peck picks up on the Catholic concept of Original Sin (A reader need not be a religious believer to follow Peck's point here.) The idea of Original Sin maintains that all humans are born with a tendency toward sinfulness, which we inherit down the generations from the first biblical parents, Adam and Eve. Then, we can overcome Original Sin through God's grace and redemption.

Scott Peck has his observational idea about Original Sin, which is not necessarily a religious one, that he drew from many hundreds of patients he had dealt with over decades. Many of his patients struggled for months or years to understand --- with his therapeutic help --- what their psychological and/or emotional roadblocks were to experiencing fuller, happier, and controlled lives. Once the necessary insights and understanding of the problems were discovered, a game plan was formulated to heal the patient. It was, of course, incumbent on the patient to work and implement the healing process. Peck observed that many would not do the work or the follow-up necessary to finally defeat their challenges. Peck contends this is due to their --- and our --- innate laziness.

Laziness is the well-trodden Path of Least Resistance. It is always easiest to do nothing, requiring no energy, thought, discipline, or work.

So, an early step toward healing is your willingness to work, to expend effort. Often, massive effort. Recognizing our inclination toward laziness can somewhat blunt its power. Identify the enemy. As stated previously, a written game plan to counter inertia and laziness is a tremendous aid.

Step 3 --- Know Your Enemy to Defeat Cancer

As the commanding general in your war on cancer, you must know your enemy, its location(s), its size, its weapons, its strengths, and its weaknesses.
*What exactly is cancer?
*What probably caused your particular cancer?
*How does cancer arise and grow?
*What environment inside you allowed the cancer to thrive?
*What feeds cancer?
*What weapons effectively kill cancer and destroy its favored environment?
*How will you know when the enemy has been wiped out?
*How do you prevent its recurrence or avoid acquiring a new cancer?

Understanding What Cancer Is?
Let's start by talking about DNA.

DNA, or deoxyribonucleic acid, is like a building blueprint

for living things. It is the instruction manual that tells cells how to grow, develop, and function. Envision DNA as a long, twisted ladder (often called a double helix) of smaller building blocks called *nucleotides*. These nucleotides are arranged in a specific sequence, and this sequence determines everything from your eye color and height to how your body processes food to create energy. DNA carries the genetic information from your parents that makes you who you are! Health problems, and possibly cancer, arise when your DNA is damaged.

DNA Damage – The Usual Suspects

Cellular DNA can be damaged by various mechanisms, including:

***Environmental toxins**. Exposure to certain environmental toxins and carcinogens, such as chemicals, radiation, air & water pollutants, herbicides like Roundup and Paraquat, and pesticides can directly damage mitochondria.

***Dietary factors**. A poor diet, particularly one high in processed sugars and unhealthy fats, contributes to mitochondrial damage. Seyfried advocates for a ketogenic diet to reduce this risk, as ketones are a more efficient and less damaging fuel source for mitochondria.

***Metabolic stress**: Conditions like obesity, diabetes, and metabolic syndrome (a cluster of adverse medical conditions) can put additional stress on mitochondria, leading to dysfunction over time.

***Radiation**. UV light, X-rays, and gamma rays can cause breaks in the DNA strands or create harmful molecules (free radicals) that damage DNA.

***Biological agents**. Viruses and bacteria can integrate their DNA into host cells or produce toxins that harm DNA.

***Replicative errors**. Mistakes during DNA replication can lead to mismatches or structural abnormalities.

***Oxidative stress**. High levels of Reactive Oxygen Species

(ROS) --- highly reactive molecules containing oxygen that are natural byproducts of cellular metabolism --- can damage DNA and proteins.

***Inflammation**. Inflammation is the body's natural response to injury, infection, or harmful stimuli. This involves activating the immune system to fight to overcome and quell the aggravated inflammation site.   When the immune system loses the battle, persistent chronic inflammation can be a critical factor in damaging DNA and creating a microenvironment conducive to tumor development and growth. Conditions such as obesity and metabolic syndrome can exacerbate inflammation.

***Internal (as opposed to external) factors**. Normal cellular processes, such as the action of particular enzymes or the natural breakdown of cellular components, can inadvertently cause DNA damage.

***Genetic factors**. While genetic mutations are secondary in cancer development, some inherited genetic mutations can predispose DNA damage.

The Possible Results of DNA Damage

When the DNA is damaged, this can lead to a variety of problems for the cell and the organism as a whole, and possibly lead to cancer development. Here are some key points about what can happen to injured DNA:

***Repair mechanisms damage.** Cells have built-in repair systems that try to fix the damage. These can recognize and repair various types of damage, like broken strands or mismatched bases. With severe DNA damage, cell repair may not happen.

***Apoptosis interruption**. If the damage to its DNA is too great and cannot be repaired, the cell might undergo *apoptosis*, which is normally a controlled process of cell death. This prevents damaged cells from dividing and potentially causing issues. However, when naturally healthy and normal apoptosis death does not take place, the DNA-damaged "Frankenstein" cell (hereafter Franken cell) survives, cheating death.

***Mutations.** If the cell damage isn't repaired correctly, it can lead to mutations and changes in the DNA sequence. Some mutations may be harmless, while other Franken cells can lead to diseases, including cancer.

***Cell dysfunction.** Damaged DNA can impair a cell's ability to function correctly, affecting processes like normal growth, division, and response to signals from other cells.

***Accelerated aging.** Accumulated DNA damage over time is linked to accelerated aging and age-related diseases, like cancer, as cells lose their ability to function effectively.

Overall, DNA damage can disrupt normal cellular processes and possibly give rise to Franken cells and cancer.

Cancer's Beginning

A *gene* is a unit of heredity that is passed from parents to their offspring. It contains the instructions necessary to build and maintain an organism's cells and pass traits to the next generation. Genes are made up of DNA.

Cancer begins when cells acquire mutations (alterations or modifications) in their genes --- made up of DNA --- that control normal cell growth, division, and death. These mutations can be caused by various factors such as environmental carcinogens, diet, lifestyle habits, diseases like obesity and diabetes, infections, chronic inflammation, radiation, viruses, inherited genetics, or random errors during DNA replication.

These mutated cells --- Franken cells --- affect vital regulatory *genes*, particularly *proto-oncogenes*, which promote normal cell growth, and tumor suppressor genes, which inhibit excessive cell growth. When these genes are altered/damaged, cells lose their healthy growth control mechanisms.

As a result of these genetic changes, cancer cells begin to divide and multiply rapidly without responding to the standard signals and commands that regulate and control natural cell growth and death. Cancer that starts in the body's tissues and organs becomes a tumor. As cancer cells grow, spread, and invade organs and tissues, it will disrupt the natural and essential functions of these organs and tissues. A cancerous liver, heart, pancreas, kidneys, thyroid, or stomach will cease to function correctly and eventually kill the host.

An example of a cancer not creating solid tumors would be leukemias, cancers of blood cells that produce many abnormal cancerous blood cells that circulate throughout the body, disrupting oxygen, nutrients, T-cells, and essential hormone transport.

Resourceful cancer cells often develop the ability to avoid normal programmed cell death (apoptosis), allowing them to survive and continue dividing when they should typically die.

Another mechanism by which cancer spreads is through *angiogenesis*, a condition whereby cancerous tissues grow by stimulating the formation of new blood vessels to supply oxygen and nutrients to the growing mass, further supporting their rapid growth.

If a cancer tumor remained entirely confined within a single, one-location-only mass, it could be removed by surgery or killed by focused radiation or other target-specific treatments. Unfortunately, cancer has evolved to eventually spread --- *metastasize* --- to different locations, invading other tissues and systems.

As nomadic cancer cells acquire the ability to break away from the original tumor site to invade new lands, they travel through the bloodstream and lymph system to relocate and grow in surrounding tissues and spread to other parts of the body --- the liver, pancreas, lung, heart, stomach, et al. The lethality of the cancer has now increased exponentially when it metastasizes. At this point, the cancer infection is referred to as "Stage 4," typically a death sentence if left untreated.

A Closer View of Identifying the Enemy and Its Strengths

Sun Tzu emphasizes the importance of understanding the enemy in his book *The Art of War*: "If you know the enemy and know yourself, you need not fear the result of a hundred battles."

According to **Dr. Jason Fung**, in his book *The Cancer Code*, there are 8 hallmarks shared by all cancer types. These hallmarks provide a framework for understanding how cancer cells operate, evade healthy regulatory mechanisms, and spread. Here's a brief explanation of each hallmark, noting cancer's defining abilities:

1. Sustaining proliferative signaling. Cancer cells can continuously signal themselves or nearby cells to grow and divide at an accelerated rate, bypassing the standard mechanisms that regulate orderly cell growth.

2. Evading growth suppressors: Tumors develop ways to ignore/outwit healthy signals that would typically stop cell division, such as tumor suppressor genes.

3. Resisting cell death: Cancer cells can evade *apoptosis* (programmed cell death), allowing these Franken cells to survive longer than normal cells, even in conditions that would usually trigger cell death.

4. Enabling replicative immortality: Cancer cells adapt the abilities to replicate and grow indefinitely.

5. Inducing angiogenesis: Tumors can stimulate the formation of new blood vessels --- *angiogenesis* --- to supply the growing tumor with nutrients and oxygen, which is critical for their growth and survival.

6. Activating invasion and metastasis: Cancer cells can spread --- metastasize --- to other parts of the body by invading surrounding tissues and entering the bloodstream or lymphatic system, forming additional secondary tumors.

7. Deregulating cellular energetics: Cancer cells often alter their metabolism to support rapid growth, favoring processes like anaerobic glycolysis respiration even in the presence of oxygen (the Warburg effect) instead of normal, healthy oxidative phosphorylation.

8. Avoiding immune destruction: Cancerous tumors can develop mechanisms to evade detection and attack by the immune system, allowing them to grow and proliferate without being eliminated by healthy immunity defenses. Fung writes that cancer cells are a reversion to an earlier cellular evolutionary format, the unicellular or single-cell organism, compared to a multicellular organism with its many, many diverse cells that form the tissues and organs that all work together for its growth, maintenance, and function. Cancer already exists inside every cell of every multicellular organism, according to Fung. The dormant cancer cell, then, needs only to be awakened or activated by DNA injury, mitochondria damage, a genetic trigger, or other means mentioned. When the natural cancer suppressors --- such as p53 genes, T cells, interferon, and CTLA-4 proteins --- which typically keep cancer cells in check in a healthy organism, are weakened or disabled, the cancer thrives, grows, and spreads.

Harboring the Enemy --- What Environmental, "Fertile Soil" Conditions in the Body Allow Cancer to Grow, and What Feeds It?

Once cancer is established in the body, certain factors contribute to its growth and sustenance. Here's a look at what "feeds" or creates an environment that supports an established cancer tumor. To destroy the supportive environment and starve the cancer, the patient or advocate must know these adaptions and how they can be disrupted or terminated.

1. Blood supply expansion. Tumors often stimulate the formation of new blood vessels through a process called *angiogenesis*. These new vessels provide the tumor with oxygen and nutrients, which are crucial for its growth and survival.

2. Cancer food. Cancer-feeding nutrients include:

a. Glucose. Cancer cells are known for their high glucose consumption. They rely on glucose for energy and growth, often exhibiting increased glycolysis even in the presence of oxygen, a phenomenon known as the Warburg effect. Excessive sugar, refined carbohydrates, and processed foods in the American diet feed cancer.

b. Amino Acids. Tumors also require amino acids, like glutamine, for protein synthesis and other metabolic processes. Some tumors can even modify the local environment to increase the availability of these essential nutrients. Amino acids such as glycine and serine, for instance, promote the growth of lymphoma and intestinal cancers, suggesting that diets restricting these could potentially slow cancer growth.

3. Hormones. Certain cancers, like breast and prostate cancer, are influenced by hormones. For example, estrogen and progesterone can encourage the growth of breast cancer cells that have hormone receptors, while androgen hormones can stimulate prostate cancer.

4. Growth factors. Tumors can produce their own "growth factors" or modify their environment to secrete factors that promote their growth and spread. These growth factors are molecules that enhance cancer's survival. In normal cells, growth factors are regulated and support healthy tissue growth and repair. Cancer cells, however, can manipulate them to their benefit.

5. Immune system interaction. Tumors can evade the immune system through various mechanisms, such as producing immune-suppressive factors or altering their cells' surface markers. This allows them to continue growing without being attacked by healthy immune cells. Lifestyle choices, diet, stress, radiation, and chemotherapy, among other factors, can weaken the immune system.

6. Microenvironment encouragement. A *stoma* is an opening in the body that allows for the passage of body or cell waste. The tumor-encouraging microenvironment, including surrounding connective tissue, immune cells, and extracellular matrix, can support tumor growth. Tumors can modify a stroma, the exit for waste products, to create a supportive growth environment for cancer.

7. Chronic inflammation. Tumors often thrive in an inflammatory environment. Inflammation is the body's immune response trying to fight off or heal an infection or injury. Chronic inflammation can promote tumor growth by providing growth factors and suppressing immune system responses that target cancer cells.

8. Metabolic waste. Tumors can utilize the waste products from other cells to create energy. For example, lactate, a byproduct of anaerobic metabolism, can be taken up by cancer cells and used for energy.

9. Aberrant cell signaling pathways. Many cancers have mutations or alterations in signaling pathways that control cell growth, division, and survival. These pathways can be hijacked by cancer cells to support their development.

10. Genetic mutations. Mutations in *oncogenes*, genes that promote cell growth, or tumor suppressor genes, genes that inhibit cell growth, can drive uncontrolled tumor growth. These mutations can influence how tumors acquire nutrients and grow.

Knowing how to counteract and attack these ten cancer-promoting factors will be part of your Master Battle Plan.

A Useful Cancer Perspective from Dr. Thomas Seyfried

From an interview on YouTube entitled "This Is Feeding Cancer Cells!" Seyfried says, "Every major cancer that I have studied has defects in the number, structure, and function of the *mitochondria* (the organelle in the cell that produces energy). This causes the cell to fall back on a primitive form of energy (and energy production), which is *fermentation* (respiration and energy production not requiring oxygen), and this leads to unregulated cell growth," a hallmark of cancer.

Metabolism and Metabolic Disease

Here are some essential concepts for explaining Seyfried's view of cancer as a *metabolic disease.*

Metabolism is the set of life-sustaining chemical reactions in your body that help convert food into energy, build and repair tissues, and manage waste products.

A *metabolic disease* happens when these processes don't work correctly. This can be due to genetic defects, lifestyle factors, environmental toxins, or other underlying health conditions like obesity and diabetes.

Common metabolic diseases include diabetes (where the body struggles to handle sugar), thyroid disorders (affecting metabolism speed), obesity (a chronic energy imbalance, where caloric intake exceeds caloric expenditure), and inherited conditions like phenylketonuria (PKU), where the body cannot break down specific proteins properly.

Symptoms can vary widely depending on the specific disease but often include fatigue, weight changes, and other health issues related to improper energy use or storage. Managing metabolic diseases usually involves a combination of medication, diet, lifestyle changes, and regular monitoring by healthcare professionals.

Cancer cells with damaged *mitochondria* (the cell's energy producers) exhibit uncontrolled growth and division. This is partly due to their altered *metabolism*, which now supports rapid cell division and the ability to thrive in low-oxygen environments where fermentation respiration occurs.

Seyfried emphasizes the importance of viewing cancer as a metabolic disease rather than the traditional genetic model for several compelling reasons. He suggests that genetic mutations commonly associated with cancer are secondary effects resulting from the initial mitochondrial damage. These genetic mutations do not drive cancer but are rather consequences of metabolic changes. The metabolic shift and mitochondrial dysfunction lead to genomic instability, which results in the genetic mutations commonly observed in cancer cells. These mutations are seen as a downstream effect rather than the primary cause.

Let's consider the difference between a *genetic disease* and a *metabolic disease*.

A genetic disease is caused by abnormalities in an individual's DNA, including mutations in single genes, multiple genes, chromosomal changes, or complex interactions between genes and the environment. A genetic predisposition to a disease can be inherited from one or both parents or occur when new cell mutations arise spontaneously, creating diseases like cancer. Statistically, however, cancers from inherited genes or the result of mere random chance are relatively few. There must be another explanation: mitochondrial dysfunction, an issue of metabolism.

Seyfried makes his case for the vast majority of cancers as *metabolic diseases*, a condition that disrupts normal metabolism — the process by which your body converts food into energy and builds or breaks down substances.

Defective metabolism can affect how the body processes nutrients, resulting in functional, disease-causing issues:

***Impaired energy production.** Problems arise in converting carbohydrates, fats, or proteins into energy in the cell.

***Accumulation of toxins.** There is now an inability to break down certain potentially toxic substances, leading to harmful buildups of carcinogenic toxins in the body.

***Hormonal imbalances.** Disruptions in essential hormones, like insulin, that regulate metabolism arise and encourage cancer.

Mitochondria are key players in understanding cancer. These are the energy-producing organelles in the cell. It is here that the body's energy is produced—specifically, Seyfried views cancer as fundamentally a disease of energy metabolism and mitochondrial dysfunction.

With abundant oxygen available, o*xidative phosphorylation* is the usual metabolic process that occurs in mitochondria as the primary mechanism by which cells generate ATP, the main energy currency of the cell. When the cell's mitochondria function properly, they generate energy for the cell and the body through respiration, a multi-stage process involving the transport of oxygen to the cells where glucose is broken down to create energy. Mitochondria utilize oxygen to break down glucose to produce ATP (adenosine triphosphate), the cell's primary energy source, which then powers essential cellular activities and healthy functions, thus powering our bodies with energy.

Mitochondrial dysfunction, however, leads to a shift away from oxidative phosphorylation --- a crucial step in cell respiration using oxygen --- to *glycolysis* energy production, a process not requiring oxygen, referred to as an *anaerobic* state. Glycolysis can occur in and power Franken cells even in the presence of oxygen, a phenomenon known as the Warburg Effect. The preference of cancer cells for glycolysis over oxidative phosphorylation not only alters energy production but also changes the metabolic landscape of the cell. Cancer cells can now adapt their metabolism to support rapid growth and proliferation, utilizing various nutrients, like amino acids and fatty acids, for energy and building blocks for rapid cell division.

The metabolic alterations in cancer cells lead to supportive changes in the tumor's immediate small-scale surroundings, its microenvironment. Seyfried concludes the ability of cancer cells to metastasize (spread to other tissues and organs) is linked to their altered metabolism and respiration, using alternative mitochondrial energy production methods.

Cancer Is Created When . . . Seyfried

Utilizing the information in his research and the research studies of others, Seyfried maintains that cancer begins with damage to the cell mitochondria.

How are mitochondria injured? The same ways DNA is damaged: Reactive Oxygen Species (ROS) molecules, chronic inflammation, environmental toxins, poor diet, radiation, cell replication errors, certain viruses and bacteria, metabolic stress, and occasionally genetic factors.

Cancer develops and grows when the injured mitochondria switch from normal oxygen-based respiration (oxidative phosphorylation) to produce energy to anaerobic *fermentation* respiration (glycolysis).

Imagine your body needs energy like a car needs fuel. Your body has two main ways to get this energy: normal oxygen respiration or undesirable fermentation.

Normal oxygen respiration is like using high-quality, efficient fuel in your car. It happens in your cells when there's plenty of oxygen available, like when you're breathing normally. Your cells break down food (like sugars) completely, using oxygen to produce energy and making carbon dioxide and water as waste products. It's efficient and provides a lot of energy.

Fermentation is like using a less efficient, makeshift fuel when there's not enough oxygen around, like when you're out of good fuel and have to use a substitute. Your mitochondria then break down food without much oxygen, which is less efficient and doesn't produce as much energy. This creates different waste products, like lactic acid in your muscles, which can make them feel sore, or alcohol and carbon dioxide in yeast, similar to the fermentation that makes bread rise and converts sugar to alcohol and produces carbonation in beer making.

So, in simple terms, normal cell respiration is the high-efficiency, oxygen-based process that gives you lots of energy. At the same time, fermentation is a backup process that kicks in when there's not enough oxygen, which is less efficient and produces different waste products. When the mitochondria are injured, cancer utilizes the less desirable fermentation respiration.

Cancer cells with damaged mitochondria (the cell's energy producers) exhibit uncontrolled growth and division. This is partly due to their altered metabolism, which now supports rapid cell division and the ability to thrive in low-oxygen environments where fermentation respiration occurs.

Cancer cells can develop mechanisms to evade death, allowing them to survive longer than normal cells --- striving for Frankenstein immortality --- accumulate further mutations and multiply out of control.

Franken cells can modify their surrounding environment to support their growth and spread to surrounding tissues and distant body parts through the bloodstream or lymphatic system to expand the battlefield with a growing army of Franken cells. This field maneuver is called *metastasis*, potentially deadly Stage 4 cancer.

Effective Weapons Development --- The Importance of Approaching Cancer as a Metabolic Disease

Seyfried emphasizes the importance of viewing cancer as a metabolic disease rather than the traditional genetic model for compelling reasons:

1. New therapies. Understanding cancer as a metabolic disease allows for the exploration and development of non-toxic metabolic therapies. For example, dietary interventions like the ketogenic diet can restrict the energy supply to cancer cells, potentially reducing tumor growth without the harsh side effects of traditional treatments like chemotherapy and radiation.

2. Holistic approaches. By focusing on metabolic health, holistic strategies can be developed for cancer prevention and management. This might include lifestyle and dietary changes that promote metabolic balance, such as controlling blood sugar levels, reducing inflammation, and improving mitochondrial function.

3. Addressing the cause. Viewing cancer through a metabolic lens shifts the focus from merely treating symptoms to addressing underlying causes. This approach aims to correct the metabolic imbalances and mitochondrial dysfunctions that may contribute to the onset and progression of cancer, potentially leading to more effective and long-lasting solutions.

4. Prioritizing metabolic health. While genetic mutations must be taken into account, Dr. Seyfried argues that metabolic dysregulation is what often precedes genetic mutations. By prioritizing metabolic health, it may be possible to prevent the mutations from occurring in the first place or limit their impact.

5. Prompting new research. The metabolic perspective drives new research directions and innovative discoveries. By studying the metabolic processes of cancer cells, researchers can uncover novel targets for treatment, leading to potential breakthroughs that might have been overlooked under the traditional genetic paradigm, where only chemotherapy, radiation, and immunotherapy drugs are used.

Functional medicine experts like Dr. Mark Hyman, Dr. Peter Attia, Dr. Jason Fung, and Dr. Joseph Mercola, mentioned in this book, agree with Seyfried's view and shape their cancer-fighting approaches from a metabolic disease perspective.

A Final Note from Our Understanding of Cancer

As a preview of one obvious treatment approach --- starving cancer --- let's consider what some of our experts have to say about a couple of obvious causal factors as we seek to treat and prevent the recurrence of cancer.

Cancer cells rely heavily on glucose (sugar) and glutamine, an amino acid, for energy and growth through a process called glycolysis, even in the presence of oxygen (the Warburg effect). The dysfunctional mitochondria in cancer cells lead to a shift towards fermentation metabolism, which feeds cancer growth.

Standard cancer treatments for mainstream Western medicine practitioners include surgery, chemotherapy, and radiation. Too often, these fail to stop the cancer and save the life of the patient while not addressing obvious and effective alternative treatments.

According to the American Cancer Society, in 2022, 17 million Americans --- 1 in 20 people --- were afflicted with cancer. In 2023, almost 2 million Americans were newly diagnosed with cancer, and 609,000+, the population of Detroit, died. Only heart disease kills more Americans in a year.

Dr. Thomas Seyfried and our other cited experts emphasize a comprehensive, holistic strategy that targets the metabolic dependencies of cancer cells, aiming to starve them by depriving them of their primary energy sources while supporting overall patient health and resilience. This broad and inclusive approach may eliminate the need for, or a complement to, the standard treatments of surgery, chemotherapy, and radiation.

Of course, diet is a massive first line component of a holistic cancer treatment approach.

Dr Thomas Seyfried estimates that **diet** and metabolic issues could be implicated in up to 70% of cancers. Source: Seyfried, Thomas N., *Cancer as a Metabolic Disease: On the Origin, Management, and Prevention of Cancer.*

Dr. Leigh Erin Connealy has stated that "70-90% of cancers are linked to **diet and lifestyle** factors." This quote can be found in her book *The Cancer Revolution: A Groundbreaking Program to Restore Your Health.*

Dr. Joseph Mercola, in his book *The No-Grain Diet,* states,

"Up to 70% of cancers could be prevented through **dietary and lifestyle** changes."

Dave Asprey states in his *The Metabolic Approach to Cancer* that "Research has repeatedly shown that 95 percent of cancer cases are directly linked to **diet and lifestyle**."

Dr. Mark Hyman states in *Food: What the Heck Should I Eat?* "At least 40% of cancers are related to **diet and lifestyle** factors."

Armed with knowing this agreed-upon list of some major causal factors for the development and growth of cancer --- with diet and lifestyle as universal factors cited here --- you can control what you eat while staying optimally hydrated and physically active to starve The Enemy. Though not your only weapon of war, this is a logical, noninvasive starting point. Of course, this will be one of your strategies written into your Master Battle Plan in Step 7.

Step 4 --- Determine What May Have Caused Your Cancer to Customize Your Specific Treatments

Dr. Mark Hyman is a leading advocate of functional medicine, which focuses on **identifying and addressing the root causes of disease**, not merely treating the disease symptoms. Part of effective treatment and the prevention of the recurrence of a particular cancer is to know what caused it and its source. Cancer is rarely a random event. Find the cause to target your specific cancer and possibly find the cure.

He suggests that while conventional medicine is good at "cutting it, burning cancer, and poisoning it with surgery, radiation, and drugs," many doctors fail to treat or understand the root cause of cancer. However, he also states, that "once you have cancer, an integrated approach of chemo, radiation, and surgery, combined with boosting your immune system and creating an inhospitable environment for cancer, is critical."

Hyman emphasizes a comprehensive approach to understanding the underlying causes of an individual's cancer. Here are some steps he typically suggests:

1. Comprehensive Medical History: Review your medical history, including your family history of cancer and other diseases, to identify patterns and risk factors.

2. Lifestyle Assessment: Evaluate your lifestyle factors such as diet, physical activity, stress levels, and sleep patterns, as these can significantly impact health.

3. Environmental Exposures: Identifying potential environmental toxins or exposures that may contribute to cancer risk, such as chemicals, heavy metals, or radiation.

4. Genetic Testing: Consider genetic testing to determine if there are inherited mutations that increase your cancer risk, which can guide your prevention and treatment strategies.

5. Nutritional Evaluation: Assessing your nutritional status and dietary habits, as nutrition plays a crucial role in cancer development and recovery.

6. Gut Health Analysis: Explore your gut health and microbiome balance, as imbalances can influence inflammation and immune function.

7. Emotional and Mental Health Check: Consider the possible psychological aspects, including stress and trauma, which can affect your overall health and well-being.

These tests and research items can take much time and effort but can be life-and-death crucial. Vow to dedicate the necessary work to a winning battle plan.

The case for understanding the root cause of a patient's cancer to more precisely and effectively treat it is supported by reputable scientific studies. Here are three:

*A landmark study published in *The New England Journal of Medicine* (Slamon et al., 2001) found that breast cancer patients with HER2 gene amplification showed significant improvement in survival rates when treated with trastuzumab. This research emphasized the importance of genetic profiling to understand the cancer's root cause – its *etiology* --- in selecting effective targeted therapies.

*Lung cancer can have a variety of causes. A study published in *Cancer Research* (Kris et al., 2014) demonstrated that lung cancer patients with a history of tobacco use exhibited distinct tumor profiles. This differentiation allowed for the development of tailored treatment strategies, resulting in improved outcomes for smokers receiving personalized care based on their cancer's specific etiology.

*A study published in *The Lancet* (Kitchener et al., 2009) revealed that identifying the presence of HPV (Human Papilloma Virus) in cervical cancer patients facilitated more effective vaccination strategies and treatment protocols. This targeted approach significantly reduced recurrence rates among HPV-related cervical cancer patients.

Step 5 --- Destroying the Fertile Ground on Which Cancer Grows

Creating Fertile Ground: Key factors and conditions associated with an increased risk of getting cancer

As stated before, acquiring cancer is not a random event. There is a cause, sometimes multiple causes. Knowing the causal factors and conditions can prevent cancer in the first place, aid in its defeat and healing once infected, and assist in preventing its recurrence. Here are recurrent themes presented by our experts about the creation of the body's "fertile ground" for growing cancer:

1. Diet. Poor diet is linked to about 30-35% of cancer deaths. The World Cancer Research Fund/American Institute for Cancer Research (2018) published a study to confirm these numbers, and the American Cancer Society (ACS) agrees, as published in their 2020 dietary guidelines for cancer prevention. Diets high in red and processed meats and unhealthy fats and low in fruits and vegetables can increase the risk of colorectal, breast, prostate, and pancreatic cancers, among others. According to functional medicine physician Dr. Mark Hyman, 70% of cancers are diet related. "The thing I really focus on around diet is starch and sugar because we know that insulin resistance, pre-diabetes, diabetes, and belly fat create a cancer-causing factory. " (Hyman is the Head of Strategy and Innovation at the prestigious Cleveland Clinic Center for Functional Medicine and the founder and director of The UltraWellness Center, a functional medicine practice in Massachusetts. He has written several best-selling books on health and wellness, including *The Blood Sugar Solution 10-Day Detox Diet, Eat Fat, Get Thin, The UltraMind Solution,* and *Food: What the Heck Should I Eat?*)

2. Obesity and being overweight. A stunning 42% of Americans are obese, including 19% of children aged 18 and under. Being overweight or obese increases the risk of cancer, including breast (post-menopause), colorectal, and endometrial cancers, among others. Obesity can affect hormone levels and inflammatory pathways that can contribute to cancer development, too. Fat tissue can produce hormones and other substances that encourage cancer growth.

3. Physical inactivity. Lack of physical activity is associated with an increased risk of several cancers, including breast, colon, and endometrial cancers. Regular exercise helps maintain a healthy weight and reduces cancer risk and other diseases.

4. Chronic dehydration. Excluding the bones, body tissues and organs are typically 70% - 90% water. Staying adequately hydrated is crucial to a healthy body. While not commonly listed as a direct cause of cancer, this condition can contribute to various health issues that might indirectly impact cancer risk. Adequate hydration is crucial for maintaining cellular function and DNA integrity. Persistent dehydration can lead to cellular stress and damage, which might potentially increase the risk of mutations and cancer over time. Also, the immune system's crucial defense function is impaired, which affects the body's ability to detect and destroy cancer cells.

5. Smoking is one of the leading causes of cancer, responsible for approximately 25-30% of cancer deaths. It is particularly associated with lung cancer but also contributes to cancers of the mouth, throat, esophagus, pancreas, bladder, and more. The carcinogens in tobacco smoke damage the DNA in cells, leading to cancer.

6. Human Papillomavirus (HPV). Certain strains of HPV are strongly linked to cervical cancer, as well as cancers of the anus, penis, and throat. HPV can cause changes in the cells that may lead to cancer.

7. Particular infections are significant cancer risk factors. Human papillomavirus (HPV) is linked to cervical cancer, hepatitis B and C to liver cancer, and Helicobacter pylori to stomach cancer. Infections account for about 15-20% of cancers worldwide. These viral infections are major risk factors for liver cancer. They cause chronic inflammation and damage to the liver, which can lead to cancer over time.

8. Excessive Alcohol Consumption. Alcohol is a chemical carcinogen that contributes to cancers. It accounts for about 3.5% of cancer deaths globally. Regular and heavy alcohol use is a risk factor for several types of cancer, including breast, liver, esophagus, and colorectal cancer. Alcohol can also increase the risk of cancer by causing inflammation and oxidative stress, factors in cell mutation.

9. Asbestos exposure is a known cause of mesothelioma, a rare form of cancer that affects the lining of the lungs, abdomen, or heart. Found as a construction material in older homes and buildings, it can also increase the risk of lung cancer.

10. Excessive UV radiation from the sun or tanning beds is a leading cause of skin cancer, including melanoma, squamous cell carcinoma, and basal cell carcinoma. UV radiation can damage the DNA in skin cells, causing some to mutate.

11. Radiation exposure, including x-rays. High levels of ionizing radiation, such as that from radiation therapy for other cancers, x-rays, radon gas, or radiation released during nuclear accidents, like Chornobyl and Fukushima, can increase the risk of developing cancers like leukemia and thyroid cancer.

12. Farming and industrial chemicals. Prolonged exposure to certain chemicals, such as benzene and formaldehyde, and some pesticides and herbicides, like Roundup and Paraquat, can increase cancer risk. These chemicals can act as carcinogens or cause cellular damage that leads to cancer.

13. Hormonal factors. Hormonal imbalances and hormone replacement therapies can influence the risk of cancers such as breast, ovarian, and prostate cancers

14. Genetic mutations and inherited syndromes. Some cancers are caused by inherited genetic mutations or genetic syndromes, such as BRCA1 and BRCA2 mutations (associated with breast and ovarian cancer) or Lynch syndrome (related to colorectal cancer). These genetic factors can significantly increase the risk of certain cancers and are often triggered by environmental toxins and lifestyle choices, such as poor diet, obesity, inflammation, and too little physical activity.

Please note that genetic causes of cancer --- often, apparently, thought to be the primary cause by many Western medicine traditionalists --- are only one possibility of many possible causes. In my research, the National Cancer Institute (NCI), American Cancer Society (ACS), Mayo Clinic, Cancer Research UK, and the National Institute of Health (NIH) ALL maintain that genetic factors account for no more than 10% of cancers. So this means that at least 90% --- 9 out of 10 --- cancers have non-genetic causes. Again, it is imperative to know and discover the cause to effectively treat your cancer and prevent its return.

How do we destroy the supportive environment --- the Fertile Ground --- and aid in killing the cancer?

Addressing each of the ten contributors mentioned in *Step 3 – Know Your Enemy to Defeat Cancer* --- that allow a cancer tumor to survive and thrive involves a variety of strategies, many of which are incorporated into current cancer treatments and research. Here's how each of the ten factors can potentially be neutralized to starve or inhibit a cancer tumor.

1. Blood supply and angiogenesis inhibitors. Drugs known as angiogenesis inhibitors can block the formation of new blood vessels that tumors need for growth. Examples include bevacizumab (Avastin) and sunitinib (Sutent). These agents target vascular endothelial growth factor (VEGF) or other factors involved in angiogenesis.

2. Nutrient and dietary approaches:
*Targeting glucose metabolism. Start by limiting or eliminating sugar, refined carbohydrates, and processed foods. There are drugs that inhibit glycolysis or glucose uptake, which can potentially starve cancer cells of the energy they need. For instance, 2-deoxy-D-glucose (2-DG) is a compound being studied for its ability to interfere with glucose metabolism in cancer cells.

*Amino acid deprivation. Certain therapies aim to reduce the availability of essential amino acids. For example, drugs like L-asparaginase deplete asparagine, an amino acid necessary for some leukemia cells.

3. Hormone therapies. For hormone-dependent cancers, such as breast or prostate cancer, hormone therapies can be used to block hormone production or action. Tamoxifen and aromatase inhibitors are example therapies for breast cancer, while anti-androgens like enzalutamide are used for prostate cancer.

4. Growth factors and inhibitors of growth factor signaling. Targeted therapies can inhibit the signaling pathways activated by growth factors. For example, drugs like erlotinib (Tarceva) inhibit the epidermal growth factor receptor (EGFR) pathway, which is involved in some cancers.

5. Immune system interactions:
*Strengthen your immune system with a healthy diet, adequate hydration, regular exercise, quality and adequate sleep, and stress relief techniques.
*Immunotherapy aims to enhance the body's immune response against cancer cells. Checkpoint inhibitors like pembrolizumab (Keytruda) or CAR-T cell therapies can help the immune system recognize and destroy cancer cells.
*Immune modulators. Agents like interferons can boost the immune response and aid in the recognition and elimination of cancer cells.

6. Stroma modulation. *Stroma* refers to the supportive tissue or framework of an organ or, in this case, a cancerous tumor. Drugs designed to target the tumor's stromal components can potentially destroy the tumor by disrupting its supportive stromal environment.

7. Quelling inflammation. Inflammation can encourage tumor growth, enhancing the "fertile ground" in which it grows.
*Eat anti-inflammatory foods like berries, nuts, turmeric, green leafy vegetables, and fatty fish, like salmon.
*Regular exercise, quality sleep, and adequate hydration help alleviate inflammation.
*Drugs that reduce inflammation include nonsteroidal anti-inflammatory drugs (NSAIDs) or selective COX-2 inhibitors like celecoxib have been cited for their potential role in cancer prevention and treatment. (CancerChoices.org cites

the upside of NSAIDs) And, consider corticosteroids. These drugs can reduce inflammation and are used in combination with other therapies, especially in blood and bone marrow cancers.

8. Targeting metabolic waste utilization. *Lactate* is a byproduct of anaerobic metabolism when cancer cells break down glucose for energy in the absence of oxygen and can be used to fuel a tumor. Targeting lactate metabolism or lactate transport can potentially disrupt a tumor's ability to utilize these byproducts for its growth.

9. Targeted drug therapy. Drugs that specifically disrupt cancer's abnormal *signaling pathways* can be effective. These pathways are networks of proteins and molecules that help cells communicate with each other and respond to their environment. In cancer, signaling pathways can be hijacked or mutated, leading to malignant behavior. Drugs that inhibit or block these pathways can help defeat the cancer.

10. Precision medicine. Treatments tailored to specific genetic mutations in cancer cells can be effective. For example, targeted therapy drugs like imatinib (Gleevec) are used for cancers with specific genetic mutations that cause cancer. Additionally, there are treatment innovations like CRISPR (Clustered Regularly Interspaced Short Palindromic Repeats), a revolutionary genetic engineering tool that allows scientists to precisely alter DNA within living cells. Using CRISPR in cancer treatment aims to target and kill cancer cells either directly or to enhance the body's immune response to recognize and destroy cancer.

Know and Fortify Your First Line of Defense: Your Immune System

Your body is assaulted by pathogens and toxins every second of every day, including attacks by potential cancer-causing agents. A healthy immune system naturally and wonderfully summons its soldiers to locate, fight, destroy, and remove those villainous agents that would harm or even kill you. So, your immune system's health is imperative to prevent or overcome cancer.

Ever-present health enemies that a vibrant immune system successfully locates and destroys include:

***Viruses.** Certain viruses, such as human papillomavirus (HPV) and Epstein-Barr virus (EBV), can lead to cancer. A healthy immune system typically clears these infections before they can cause harm.

***Mutated Cells**. The body regularly produces cells with DNA mutations, which have the potential to turn into cancer cells. The immune system can recognize and destroy many of these mutated cells.

***Environmental Toxins.** Agents such as tobacco smoke, asbestos, and certain chemicals. Such as glyphosate and Paraquat used in farming, can cause cancer-promoting mutations. A robust immune system helps to repair or eliminate cells before they develop into cancer.

***Radiation damage.** Exposure to ultraviolet (UV) radiation from the sun and other sources, like medical X-rays and cancer radiation treatments, can damage DNA, leading to mutations. The immune system plays a role in repairing damaged cells or eliminating them if they become dangerous.

***Bacteria.** Some bacteria, like *Helicobacter pylori*, are linked to cancer development. The healthy immune system can typically target and eradicate such infections.

Potential Immune System Damage from Radiation and Chemotherapy

If you have cancer, often your immune system has been damaged or impaired which allowed the cancer to take hold and grow. The traditionally prescribed cancer treatments of radiation and chemotherapy may further weaken the all-important immune system function. Here are some potential harmful effects of chemo and radiation:

***Bone Marrow Suppression**. Both treatments can damage the bone marrow, leading to a reduced production of white blood cells, which are crucial for the immune response.

***Lymphocyte Depletion**. Radiation and chemotherapy can decrease the number of lymphocytes (a type of white blood cell), weakening the immune system's ability to fight infections and tumors.

***Immune Cell Dysfunction**. Both treatments can impair the functionality of remaining immune cells, reducing their ability to recognize and attack harmful pathogens and abnormal cells.

***Increased Susceptibility to Infections.** Patients with a compromised immune system are more vulnerable to infections, which can be more severe and complicated to treat.

***Delayed Immune Recovery.** After either treatment, it can take a long time for the immune system to recover, leaving patients at a higher risk for opportunistic infections and other complications related to the cancer being treated.

***Chronic Inflammation**. Radiation and chemotherapy can cause chronic inflammation, which may further damage healthy tissues and damage immune function.

***Autoimmune Reactions.** In some cases, radiation and chemotherapy may trigger autoimmune reactions, where the immune system mistakenly attacks the body's healthy cells and tissues.

Knowing these potential injuries to the all-important immune system may prompt important discussions about alternative therapies to radiation and chemotherapy in your cancer war. As always, do your research and consider getting second and third opinions about cancer treatments. Prepare a list of questions. Remember: YOU are the general to prosecute the war. Doctors are your necessary soldiers, not God.

Boosting and Maintaining a Healthy Immune System – 10 Strategies

A healthy body, complemented by a healthy mind and emotional state, is successfully defended by a stellar immune system. A high-octane immune system and optimal cancer-free health are driven by some of the recurrent-theme protocols laid out by the cancer experts cited in this book. To review, see these in your written step-by-step Battlefield Master Plan, Step 7.

Your never-ending challenge is to persevere, fight your natural tendency toward laziness, and commit to do the work. These, in turn, are driven by your strong reasons for living and your Noble Purpose. The world needs you and the gifts & talents only YOU have to offer. You have a Noble Mission, General. A loving duty. Never forget.

Your immune system is your first line of defense against cancer. A healthy immune system has natural functional mechanisms that seek out and destroy cancer cells before they can accumulate, grow, and spread. You can take specific actions as part of your Master Battle Plan to boost your immune system.

All of the following activities and treatments serve to boost your cancer-fighting immune system and move you toward self-healing. You will notice recurrent themes.

1. Live with purpose and love. When individuals feel their lives have meaning, they experience less stress and anxiety. Reduced stress levels have been linked to lower cortisol levels, supporting immune function. Research published in the journal *Psychosomatic Medicine* reveals that people with a strong sense of purpose tend to have lower inflammatory markers. Reduced inflammation boosts the immune system. Also, people with a clear sense of purpose are often more motivated to maintain healthy lifestyles that support a robust immune system.

2. Maintain a Balanced Diet. Eat a variety of fruits, vegetables, whole grains, and lean proteins. Avoid sugar and processed carbohydrates. Nutrients like vitamins C, D, and E and minerals such as zinc and selenium play crucial roles in immune function.

3. Stay Hydrated. Drinking plenty of water helps your body produce lymph, which carries white blood cells and other immune system cells.

4. Regular Exercise. Engage in physical activity for at least 30 minutes a day. Exercise boosts circulation, which allows immune cells to move more effectively through the body.

5. Get Adequate Quality Sleep. Aim for 7-9 hours of quality sleep per night. Sleep is essential for producing and releasing cytokines, proteins that aid the immune response.

6. Manage Stress. Chronic stress can suppress the immune system. Practice relaxation techniques such as mindfulness, meditation, or yoga to manage stress.

7. Maintain Good Hygiene. Washing your hands regularly and properly, keeping up with vaccinations, and practicing other hygiene measures help prevent infections.

8. Avoid Smoking. Smoking weakens the immune system and makes the body less successful at fighting diseases.

9. Limit Alcohol Consumption. Excessive alcohol intake can impair the immune system. Limit it to moderate levels, like one drink a day.

10. Stay Connected. Social interactions and maintaining relationships help reduce stress and boost overall health, contributing to a stronger immune system.

Step 6 - Know What Our All-Star Researchers and Practitioners Recommend to Defeat Cancer

Dr. Thomas Seyfried's cancer prevention & treatment protocols

1. Ketogenic diet. Restrict glucose (sugar) availability and elevate ketone bodies in the blood by eating cancer-starving foods and eliminating those that feed cancer. Eat a high-fat, low-carbohydrate, and moderate-protein diet to reduce blood glucose levels and increase blood ketone levels, which cancer cells have difficulty utilizing for energy. Like healthy cells, cancer cells will die if they do not produce energy to live. Ketone Foods:

*Eggs provide a versatile source of protein and healthy fats.

*Fatty fish, particularly salmon, for its omega-3 fatty acids and protein content.

*Meat and poultry are essential for their high protein and fat content, with an emphasis on choosing quality cuts, grass-fed and free range.

*Avocados have healthy monounsaturated fats and low net carb content.

*Leafy greens such as spinach, kale, and Swiss chard are valued for their low-carb content and high nutrient density.

*Nuts and seeds, especially those lower in carbs like pecans, almonds, walnuts, Brazil nuts, and macadamia nuts, offer healthy fats and protein.

*High-fat dairy products, including cheese and butter, are keto-friendly options. As always, organic and grass-fed.

*Olive oil and olives have healthy fat content and versatility in cooking.

*Non-starchy vegetables, particularly cauliflower, kale, spinach, broccoli, and zucchini have low-carb content and versatility as substitutes for higher-carb foods.

*While not universally listed in the top 10, dark chocolate (with high cocoa content) is often mentioned as a keto-friendly treat due to its relatively low-carb content and potential health benefits. Dark chocolate (at least 70% cocoa) is packed with powerful antioxidants, such as flavonoids, polyphenols, and catechins. These compounds help protect the body against free radicals, which can cause oxidative stress and damage cells.

*What about common fruits? While fruits are generally high in carbohydrates and sugars, which can make them challenging to include in a ketogenic diet, some fruits are lower in carbs and can be enjoyed *in moderation*: strawberries, raspberries, blackberries, blueberries, coconut flesh, limes, lemons, and tomatoes.

2. Caloric restriction – excess body fat is cancer's ally.
*Lower overall calorie intake to reduce glucose availability and create an energy deficit for cancer cells.

*Controlled caloric intake, often combined with intermittent fasting, stresses and starves cancer cells metabolically. Simply, eat less. Being obese, even overweight, fuels cancer.

*Belly fat, especially when it accumulates as visceral fat around organs, can contribute to cancer progression. Shed the fat.

*Inflammation: Visceral fat releases inflammatory cytokines and adipokines, which promote chronic low-grade inflammation. This inflammation can create an environment conducive to cancer cell growth and survival. Caloric restriction can aid in decreasing inflammation.

*Visceral fat can alter hormone levels, such as increasing estrogen production, which is linked to hormone-sensitive cancers like breast and ovarian cancer. Test to discover specifics and rebalance your hormones.

*Excess belly fat often leads to insulin resistance and higher insulin levels and insulin-like growth factors (IGFs). Elevated insulin and IGFs can stimulate cancer cell proliferation and inhibit apoptosis (natural cell death), creating conditions favorable for cancer development. Start with a blood test to discover your insulin levels to bring it into balance.

*Fat tissue can affect overall metabolism, including glucose and lipid metabolism, which may influence cancer cell energy sources and growth.

*Excess fat can cause chronic inflammation and altered immune responses and can impair the body's ability to detect and destroy cancer cells.

3. Intermittent fasting. Fasting induces metabolic stress on cancer cells by depriving them of their preferred fuel sources.

*Periods of fasting followed by eating windows can enhance the effectiveness of a ketogenic diet and caloric restriction. A simple example of restricted fasting might be eating only between 8 a.m. and 5 p.m. This results in a 15-hour fasting window. Fasting can combat cancer through several mechanisms beyond calorie restriction.

*Fasting stimulates *autophagy*, a cellular process where damaged cells and components are broken down and removed. This helps eliminate dysfunctional cells, including potentially cancerous ones.

*Fasting induces *ketosis*, where the body burns fat for energy instead of glucose. Cancer cells often rely on glucose for growth, so reducing glucose availability can starve them.

*Fasting lowers insulin levels and insulin-like growth factor (IGF) levels. High insulin and IGF levels can promote cancer cell proliferation, so reducing these levels can inhibit cancer growth.

*Fasting can enhance the immune system's ability to target and destroy cancer cells. It may boost the production of certain immune cells and improve their functionality.

*Fasting triggers cellular stress responses, such as increased production of heat shock proteins, which can help protect normal cells while making cancer cells more vulnerable to treatment.

*Fasting may lower inflammation levels in the body, which can create a less favorable environment for cancer cells.
*Fasting can induce a state of *hormesis*, where normal become more resilient to stress, potentially making healthy cells more resistant to damage while at the same time impairing the development and growth of cancer cells.

4. Hyperbaric Oxygen Therapy (HBOT). Increased oxygen levels in the blood to inhibit cancer cell growth. The use of hyperbaric oxygen chambers exposes patients to high-pressure oxygen environments, which can enhance the cytotoxic effects on cancer cells when used in conjunction with ketogenic diet and fasting.

5. Use of specific supplements and drugs. The right vitamins, supplements, and drugs support metabolic therapy and target specific pathways.
*Supplements like medium-chain triglycerides (MCT oil) increase ketone production. Also, there are drugs and supplements that inhibit glycolysis and/or enhance mitochondrial function, such as the following:
*Glycolysis inhibitors include 2-Deoxy-D-glucose (2-DG), which competes with glucose for entry into cells and inhibits glycolysis by interfering with glucose metabolism. Dichloroacetate (DCA) is another compound that, while not a direct glycolysis inhibitor, can shift metabolism from glycolysis fermentation to oxidative phosphorylation (normal cellular oxygen respiration), indirectly affecting glycolytic processes.
*Recall that Seyfried views mitochondrial injury as the gateway to cancer's creation. Mitochondrial function enhancers include Metformin, a common diabetes medication that improves mitochondrial function and decreases glucose production. Resveratrol, a natural compound found in red wine, also enhances mitochondrial function and promotes cellular health. MitoQ is a mitochondrial-targeted antioxidant that improves mitochondrial function by reducing oxidative stress. Urolithin A, derived from pomegranates, is known to

enhance mitochondrial health by promoting mitophagy, the process of removing damaged mitochondria. Alpha-lipoic acid (ALA) is another supplement that supports mitochondrial function by acting as an antioxidant and participating in energy metabolism.

6. Exercise. Enhance overall metabolic health and increase the effectiveness of the ketogenic diet with regular physical activity to improve metabolic flexibility and reduce insulin levels.

7. Stress management. Techniques like meditation, yoga, and other stress-reduction practices support overall cancer treatment efficacy.

8. Regular monitoring and adjustment of body processes and chemistry. Track your metabolic markers and adjust the treatment protocol as needed. Use regular blood tests to monitor glucose and ketone levels, as well as imaging and other diagnostic tests to assess the cancer tumor response.

Dr. Jason Fung's Cancer Prevention & Treatment Protocols

1. Intermittent fasting. Dr. Fung emphasizes the potential benefits of intermittent fasting for reducing insulin levels, which may help starve cancer cells that rely on glucose for growth.

2. Low-carbohydrate ketogenic diet. Dietary changes should include lowering carbohydrate intake and potentially shift the body's metabolism to burn fat instead of glucose, which may inhibit cancer cell proliferation. Incorporate the following into your eating regimen:

*Healthy Fats: avocados, olive oil, coconut oil, nuts & seeds (e.g., almonds, walnuts, chia seeds)

*Low-Carbohydrate Vegetables: leafy greens (e.g., spinach, kale) cruciferous vegetables (e.g., broccoli, cauliflower, Brussels sprouts), zucchini, asparagus

*Protein Sources: fatty fish (e.g., salmon, mackerel), meat

(e.g., grass-fed beef, pork, chicken), eggs. full-fat dairy products (e.g., cheese, yogurt)
*Berries (in moderation): raspberries, strawberries, blackberries
*Herbs and Spices: turmeric, garlic, ginger

Fung emphasizes the importance of minimizing carbohydrate intake, particularly from sugars and grains, while focusing on whole, nutrient-dense foods to support metabolic health and potentially hinder cancer growth.

3. Caloric restriction. Limit the overall calorie intake to impact cancer cell growth and enhance the effectiveness of other cancer treatments.

4. Exercise. Regular physical activity can improve overall health, reduce inflammation, and support metabolic health, which may have a positive effect on cancer outcomes.

5. Stress reduction. Managing stress through techniques such as meditation, mindfulness, and other relaxation practices can benefit overall health and immune function.

6. Supplements. While he emphasizes a food-first approach, Fung discusses the potential role of certain supplements in supporting metabolic health. These include:
*Vitamin D: He highlights the importance of maintaining adequate vitamin D levels, as it plays a role in immune function and may help reduce cancer risk.
*Curcumin: Found in turmeric, curcumin has anti-inflammatory properties and may inhibit cancer cell growth.
*Omega-3 Fatty Acids: These essential fats, found in fish oil, may help reduce inflammation and support overall health.
*N-acetylcysteine (NAC): This supplement can support detoxification and may help protect cells from oxidative stress.
*Resveratrol: A compound found in red wine and grapes, resveratrol has been studied for its potential anti-cancer properties.
*Coenzyme Q10 (CoQ10): This antioxidant is involved in energy production in cells and may have protective effects

against cancer.

*Selenium: An essential mineral that plays a role in antioxidant defense and may help reduce cancer risk.

*Magnesium: Important for many cellular processes, magnesium deficiency has been linked to various health issues, including cancer.

7. Address insulin resistance. Since insulin resistance is linked to various cancers, addressing this condition through lifestyle changes can pay big cancer-fighting benefits.

8. Conventional treatments. Fung underscores the importance of conventional cancer treatments, such as surgery, chemotherapy, and radiation, as essential components of a comprehensive cancer treatment plan.

9. Additional cancer therapies.

*Detoxification, aimed at reducing the body's toxic load. Minimize exposure to harmful substances found in everyday products, such as pesticides, heavy metals, and chemicals in personal care products. Using saunas can encourage sweating, which may help eliminate certain toxins through the skin. Drinking plenty of water helps flush out toxins from the body and supports kidney function, which is vital for detoxification.

*Hyperbaric Oxygen Therapy (HBOT) promotes enhanced oxygen delivery to tissues and improves treatment outcomes, most often accomplished by time spent inside a hyperbaric chamber.

Dr. Mark Hyman's Cancer-Fighting Protocols

Hyman is a passionate proponent of a holistic approach to health, emphasizing the importance of diet, lifestyle, and the environment in maintaining overall wellness. In the course of a Hyman Interview on YouTube entitled "Do These Daily Things to Reduce Your Risk of Cancer," the question was posed by the interviewer: "What are 5 of the Top 10 things you can do starting today to significantly reduce the risk of getting cancer in the future?" Hyman's answer: "The two main drivers of cancer are diet and toxins." So, he recommends the following:

1. Eat a whole food, plant-based diet. Hyman cites his belief that 70% of cancers are diet related. "The thing I really focus on around diet is starch and sugar because we know that insulin resistance, pre-diabetes, diabetes, and belly fat, that is a cancer-causing factory. " Diabetes and a pre-diabetic condition drive inflammation, which, in turn, drives cancer.

He stresses the importance of eating a variety of vegetables, fruits, nuts, seeds, legumes, and healthy fats while minimizing processed foods, sugars, and industrial seed oils. He emphasizes foods that are rich in antioxidants, phytonutrients, and fiber, all of which can help reduce inflammation and oxidative stress—two factors that contribute to cancer development.

Eat anti-inflammatory foods: berries, avocados, green tea or extract, dark chocolate, nuts (almonds, walnuts, cashews), extra virgin olive oil, turmeric curcumin, tomatoes, ginger, Omega-3 fatty acids sources (salmon, mackerel, sardines, Omega-3 supplements), spinach, kale, leafy greens, cabbage, (NOT iceberg lettuce), red or purple grapes, bell peppers, mushrooms, selenium, and pineapple.

2. Reduce environmental toxins exposure. Hyman says that in the last century, humans have been exposed to 80,000 new chemicals, very few of which have been tested for safety. Many used in the US are banned in other countries around the world. Some examples:

*Paraquat: This highly toxic farming pesticide is linked to Parkinson's disease. It's banned in 65 countries, including China and the European Union, but still used in the US. It's highly toxic and can cause kidney damage and difficulty breathing.

*Atrazine: This deadly herbicide is commonly found in American drinking water. It was banned in the European Union in 2004 but is still approved for use in the US.

*Telone: A volatile and toxic fumigant pesticide heavily used in California but was phased out in the European Union in 2007 due to risks to humans and animals. California produces more than a third of America's vegetables and two-thirds of the country's fruits and nuts.

*Neonicotinoids: These pesticides, suspected of causing mass bee colony collapses, are banned or restricted in the European Union but still widely used in the US.

*Glyphosate: This is the active ingredient in Roundup, commonly used by homeowners to rid their lawns and gardens of weeds, a deadly toxin herbicide, is banned or restricted in several countries, including the Netherlands and Sri Lanka, and will be banned in Mexico in 2024, but remains widely used in the US. In November 2023, in a Cole County, Missouri Circuit Court, a jury awarded four plaintiffs --- 2 from Missouri, 1 from New York, and 1 from California --- a total of $1.56 billion in damages from Monsanto (now owned by the German company Bayer) when the four claimed they had all acquired non-Hodgkin's lymphoma, a cancer that starts in the lymph system, by using the herbicide Roundup.

As of early 2024, Monsanto/Bayer had reached settlements in no less than 100,000. Roundup lawsuits, paying out more than $11 billion. An estimated 40,000 lawsuits are still pending, most of which are individuals claiming Roundup has caused non-Hodgkin's lymphoma or soft tissue cancers.

Logical Questions: Why is Roundup still widely available for purchase? Why would anyone put themselves, other human beings, their children, and their pets who roam their property at risk by using Roundup on their lawns and gardens and in proximity to the crops they grow and eat?

More glyphosate notes of interest: No less than 16 countries worldwide have banned glyphosate use. These include Argentina, Brazil, Austria, Vietnam, India, Thailand, and Saudi Arabia, among others. Mexico has legislation in the works to ban glyphosate in 2024.

Editorial Note: In July 2024, I received a store flyer detailing special, low-price deals at my local discount store. One of the discounted items was Roundup. If people are not concerned enough about contaminating themselves and their children with Roundup, they should know that their beloved outdoor pets walking and frolicking in the yard are at risk of poison contamination, too.

3. Exercise to reduce inflammation and insulin resistance. Inflammation can cause cancer. Inflammation is a natural immune response to harmful "stimuli" in the body, which include injury, infection, virus, bacteria, toxins/poisons, or a serious irritation in the body. With inflammation, the immune system is conducting a war against the stimuli that cause damage or infections to tissues or organs in the body when injured and damaged cells and tissues are healing or will not heal. As the immune system continues to fight but not win and inflammation persists, pain and discomfort arise, and diseases may take hold, such as diabetes, cancer, hypertension, Alzheimer's, and heart disease.

4. Manage blood sugar and insulin levels. Hyman emphasizes the importance of balancing blood sugar and insulin levels to prevent chronic diseases, including cancer. Elevated blood sugar and insulin levels are associated with a higher risk of developing several types of cancer, particularly through mechanisms like inflammation and cellular growth stimulation. Strategies include:

*Limit processed carbs and sugars.

*Focusing on low-glycemic index foods that release sugar slowly into the bloodstream (e.g., non-starchy vegetables, whole grains).

*Incorporating intermittent fasting or time-restricted eating to give the body periods of rest and improve insulin sensitivity.

5. Get your microbiome and gut healthy. The gut microbiome plays a crucial role in immune function, inflammation, and detoxification. An unhealthy gut microbiome can contribute to chronic inflammation and a

weakened immune system, both of which can promote cancer growth. Hyman advocates for strategies that support the microbiome and reduce inflammation by doing the following:
*Whole foods diet. Focus on nutrient-dense, whole foods such as fruits, vegetables, whole grains, lean proteins, and healthy fats. Avoid processed foods, sugar, and refined carbohydrates, which can disrupt gut health.
*Increase fiber intake. Consume plenty of fiber-rich foods, particularly vegetables, fruits, legumes, and whole grains, to support the growth of beneficial gut bacteria.
*Eat fermented foods. Incorporate fermented foods like yogurt, kefir, sauerkraut, and kimchi, which are rich in probiotics, to help maintain a healthy balance of gut bacteria.
*Avoid antibiotics. These can disrupt the gut microbiome.
*Manage stress. Chronic stress can negatively impact gut health, so practicing stress management techniques like meditation, yoga, and deep breathing is crucial.
*Supplement wisely. Consider taking probiotics and other gut-supportive supplements like digestive enzymes, L-glutamine, and omega-3 fatty acids to promote gut healing.
*Eliminate food sensitivities. Identify and eliminate foods that you may be sensitive to or allergic to, as these can cause inflammation and damage the gut lining.
*Stay Hydrated: Drink plenty of water to support digestion and the health of the gut lining.
*Optimize your gut's nutrient status with vitamins and supplements. Methylation nutrients – the B vitamins and Vitamin D3

Dr. Thomas Levy's Cancer-Fighting Protocols

Thomas Levy, MD --- *Curing the Incurable* --- is a proponent of high-dose Vitamin C (ascorbic acid) to combat and prevent cancer. He has many research citations to support his contentions and makes the case that Vitamin C has very few side effects.

As an alternative to intravenous Vitamin C injections, Levy makes the case for liposomal (lie-puh-sew-mul) Vitamin C. In simple terms, a liposome is a tiny bubble made out of the same material as cell membranes, which are mainly fats (lipids). It has a water-filled center and is often used to carry drugs or other substances inside the body.

Think of it like a small delivery vehicle that can protect medicine or nutrients as they travel through the body and help deliver them directly to specific cells or tissues. This makes liposomes helpful in targeted drug delivery, especially for treatments like cancer therapy.

Vitamin C (ascorbic acid) itself is water-soluble and usually not stored well in the body, meaning it gets flushed out quickly. This means liposomal Vitamin C can pass more easily through cell membranes (which are made of fats) and deliver higher concentrations of Vitamin C into the bloodstream and tissues compared to regular water-soluble Vitamin C. So, while Vitamin C remains water-soluble, the liposomal delivery mimics some advantages of fat-soluble vitamins.

Here is a summary of Levy's suggested cancer-fighting therapies:

1. Intravenous (IV) vitamin C
*Dosage: High doses ranging from 25 to 100 grams (25,000 - 100,000 mg) per session.
*Method: Delivered directly into the bloodstream via an IV, bypassing the digestive system for maximum absorption.
*Frequency: Often recommended multiple times per week for cancer patients.
*Rationale: IV Vitamin C can reach much higher blood concentrations than oral Vitamin C, potentially generating hydrogen peroxide that may selectively kill cancer cells while sparing normal cells.

2. Oral liposomal vitamin C
*Dosage: Typically 5 to 10 grams (or higher) daily.
*Method: Encapsulated in liposomes for enhanced

absorption, making it a more effective oral option compared to regular Vitamin C.

*Rationale: Liposomal Vitamin C achieves higher absorption rates than regular oral Vitamin C, allowing more to reach the bloodstream and tissues.

3. Combine with other antioxidants. Levy suggests combining high-dose Vitamin C with other antioxidants, such as glutathione and alpha-lipoic acid, to enhance its cancer-fighting potential and reduce oxidative stress in the body. This synergistic effect can boost the immune system and further inhibit cancer cell growth.

4. Supportive therapy. Levy emphasizes the importance of continuous Vitamin C intake, whether orally or intravenously, to maintain high levels in the body.

He also promotes Vitamin C's use alongside conventional cancer treatments, believing it can improve outcomes and reduce side effects like fatigue and toxicity from chemotherapy or radiation.

5. Hydrogen peroxide effect. He highlights the idea that high-dose Vitamin C acts as a pro-oxidant in high concentrations, generating hydrogen peroxide in the body. This hydrogen peroxide can damage cancer cells, which are more vulnerable to oxidative stress than healthy cells.

These protocols are based on the idea that high levels of Vitamin C can attack cancer cells directly or enhance the body's ability to fight cancer.

Dr. Joseph Mercola's Cautions and Protocols

Mercola has been a vocal critic of traditional Western cancer treatments, highlighting several perceived shortcomings. For instance, he argues that conventional cancer therapies, such as chemotherapy and radiation, often do not address the underlying causes of cancer and may lead to significant side effects. Mercola suggests that these treatments can sometimes do more harm than good.

He promotes alternative therapies and natural remedies, claiming they can be more effective and less harmful than conventional treatments, just as Hyman and Seyfried do. This includes dietary changes, supplements, and lifestyle modifications, which he believes can enhance the body's ability to fight cancer.

He often points to the influence of the pharmaceutical industry in cancer treatment, suggesting that profit motives can overshadow patient care, arguing that this leads to a lack of transparency and an emphasis on treatments that may not be in the best interest of patients.

Mercola emphasizes the importance of prevention and early intervention through lifestyle changes, nutrition, and detoxification rather than solely relying on treatments after a cancer diagnosis. Mercola believes that many cancers can be prevented through proper diet and lifestyle choices.

He has expressed skepticism about established cancer treatment protocols, claiming they are often based on outdated or insufficient evidence. He advocates for a more individualized approach to cancer treatment that considers the unique biological makeup of each patient.

Mercola's views reflect a broader skepticism of conventional medical practices, advocating for alternative approaches prioritizing holistic health and prevention. As always, purveyors of traditional Western medicine and big pharma are critical of Mercola's healing and preventative strategies.

Here again, look for common protocol themes. Mercola's recommendations:

1. Ketogenic/low-carb diet. Mercola promotes a ketogenic diet, which is high in healthy fats and low in carbohydrates, to starve cancer cells of glucose and reduce inflammation.

2. Intermittent fasting. He recommends intermittent fasting to help the body switch to burning fat for fuel, which may inhibit cancer growth.

3. Mitochondrial health. To prevent cancer, focus on supporting mitochondrial function through diet, supplements, and lifestyle changes.

4. Emotional Freedom Techniques (EFT). Use EFT, a form of psychological acupressure, to reduce stress and emotional trauma, which Mercola believes can contribute to cancer development and hinder healing.

5. Mind-body connection. He emphasizes the importance of mental and emotional health in cancer prevention and treatment.

6. Sunlight and Vitamin D. He highlights the importance of natural sunlight exposure and Vitamin D supplementation to reduce cancer risk.

7. Clean water and air. Drink clean, filtered water and breathe clean air to reduce exposure to environmental toxins.

8. Avoid toxins, including pesticides, plastics, and other chemicals that may contribute to cancer.

Dr. Kelly Turner's Health Protocols

According to her research, here are the key factors that most cancer survivors have in common and which Dr. Turner recommends:

1. Radically change your diet. Emphasize whole, plant-based foods and reduce sugar and processed food intake.

2. Take control of your health. Actively participate in your health decisions, pursuing treatments that feel right for you.

3. Following your intuition. Trust your inner voice when it comes to health decisions and life choices.

4. Exercise and movement. Use it or lose it. Our body carries our being --- mind, emotions, and spirit --- to maximize our physical range and locational opportunities on Earth. Move.

5. Cancer-fighting herbs and supplements. Incorporate natural substances that have anti-cancer properties, such as the following:

a. Turmeric (Curcumin). Known for its powerful anti-inflammatory and antioxidant properties.

b. Green Tea Extract. Contains catechins, which may help inhibit cancer cell growth.

c. Ginger. Has anti-inflammatory and antioxidant qualities that may aid in cancer prevention.

d. Garlic: Contains compounds like allicin that have been shown to have anti-cancer effects.

e. Reishi mushrooms. Known for boosting the immune system and potentially inhibiting cancer growth.

f. Milk thistle. Contains silymarin, which is believed to have anti-cancer properties, especially for liver health.

g. Vitamin D. Deficiency in Vitamin D has been linked to several types of cancers.

h. Omega-3 fatty acids. Found in fish oils and flaxseeds, these are known to have anti-inflammatory effects.

i. Astragalus. An herb used in traditional Chinese medicine for boosting the immune system.

j. Resveratrol. Found in red grapes, it is known for its antioxidant properties.

6. Release suppressed emotions. Address and release long-held negative emotions.

7. Increase positive emotions. Cultivate feelings of joy, love, and happiness.

8. Embrace social support. Build a strong network of supportive relationships.

9. Deepen your spiritual connection. Engage in practices that foster a sense of spiritual connection or purpose.

10. Have strong reasons for living. Find compelling reasons to live and stay motivated.

Note that 7 of the 10 protocols Kelly Turner lists for cancer prevention, recovery, and health restoration are mental, emotional, and spiritual guidelines, not physical.

As I survey the list, I am drawn to consider the last protocol as the foundation on which the other nine will rest. If a person with cancer has little or no reason to live, they will be unwilling to do the work required by the other nine steps for recovery and preventing a cancer recurrence.

My freelance auto mechanic, Derek, who has lung cancer and a damaged heart, has told me he is ready to die. He said he will never change his diet, exercise, quit smoking, and stop drinking alcohol, sometimes to excess, wanting to "enjoy" his remaining days. Derek believes he has nothing and no one to live for now that his wife has died.

Dr. Peter Attia's Cancer and Health Protocols

1. Nutritional strategies. Dr. Attia emphasizes the importance of a low carbohydrate, ketogenic diet to reduce insulin and glucose levels, potentially slowing cancer cell growth. He also highlights the benefits of intermittent fasting to induce autophagy, a cellular process that helps eliminate damaged cells.

2. Exercise. Regular physical activity is crucial. Exercise enhances immune function, reduces inflammation, and can improve the body's overall resilience against diseases, including cancer. "More than any other tactical domain we discuss in this book (*Outlive*), exercise has the greatest power to determine how you will live out the rest of your life," says Attia. "Going from zero weekly exercise to just ninety minutes per week can reduce your risk of dying from all causes by 14 percent. It's very hard to find a drug that can do that."

3. Sleep. Prioritizing high-quality sleep is another cornerstone. Poor sleep habits can impair the immune system and increase inflammation, potentially increasing cancer risk.

4. Stress management. Managing stress through mindfulness, meditation, or other stress-reducing techniques is vital. Chronic stress can negatively impact immune function and increase cancer risk.

5. Screening and monitoring. Attia advocates for proactive and personalized screening strategies. Regular check-ups and advanced diagnostics can help detect cancer at an earlier, more treatable stage. Attia recommends monitoring elevated blood glucose levels to discover the possibility of insulin (a hormone) resistance, whereby the efficient conversion of glucose into energy is impaired. Attia insists that this one malfunction --- insulin resistance --- increases the possibility of getting cancer by 12-fold!

A screening test I have taken personally and highly recommend is the Galleri Test, created by and available from the Grail Company. A simple blood draw and analysis screens for 50 different cancers to reveal them long before symptoms appear.

6. Pharmacological interventions. Attia often discusses the use of specific medications and supplements that may contribute to cancer prevention, though these should always be considered in consultation with a healthcare provider.

a. Aspirin. Low-dose aspirin, due to its anti-inflammatory properties, has been

suggested for its potential role in reducing the risk of certain types of cancer.

b. Metformin. Originally a medication for Type 2 diabetes, metformin has been

studied for its potential anti-cancer benefits. It may reduce cancer risk by lowering blood sugar and insulin levels.

c. Vitamin D. Adequate vitamin D levels are essential for overall health and may

lower the risk of certain cancers. Attia often highlights the importance of maintaining optimal vitamin D levels through supplementation or sensible sun exposure.

d. Curcumin. The active compound in turmeric, curcumin, possesses anti

inflammatory and antioxidant properties that may contribute to cancer prevention.

e. Omega-3 fatty acids. Found in fish oil, omega-3s have anti-inflammatory properties that play a role in reducing cancer risk.

f. N-Acetyl Cysteine (NAC). This supplement is known for its antioxidant properties and potential to replenish intracellular glutathione, which can help in cancer prevention.

Dr. Erin Connealy's Cancer-Fighting Protocols

Here are some key alternative cancer treatments and strategies from her book *The Cancer Revolution*:

1. Nutritional therapy

*Diet. Dr. Connealy advocates for a diet rich in organic vegetables, fruits, and lean proteins while reducing processed foods, sugars, and refined carbohydrates. She emphasizes the importance of a plant-based diet for its high content of antioxidants and phytochemicals that can support the immune system and help combat cancer.

*Supplementation. She recommends various supplements that support cancer treatment and overall health, such as vitamins, minerals, and herbal remedies. Essential supplements include vitamin D, omega-3 fatty acids, and probiotics.

2. Detoxification/elimination of toxins. Connealy suggests methods for detoxifying the body, such as cleansing diets, sauna therapy, and avoiding exposure to environmental toxins. She believes reducing the body's toxic burden can help improve overall health and support cancer treatment.

3. Boost immunity. Strategies to enhance immune function are central to her approach. This includes the use of supplements like medicinal mushrooms (e.g., reishi and shitake), which have immune-boosting properties.

4. Stress reduction. Connealy emphasizes the role of stress management in cancer treatment. Meditation, yoga, and mindfulness are recommended to help reduce stress and improve emotional well-being.

5. Acupuncture and massage therapy. These therapies are suggested to support symptom management and improve quality of life. Acupuncture can help with pain relief, nausea, and fatigue, while massage can aid in relaxation and stress reduction.

6. Exercise. Regular physical activity is recommended to support overall health and well-being. Exercise can help maintain a healthy weight, reduce inflammation, and improve mood and energy levels.

7. Address hormonal imbalances. For cancers that are hormone-sensitive (like breast cancer), Connealy discusses the importance of balancing hormones through diet, lifestyle changes, and possibly supplementation.

8. Advanced testing and diagnostics. Connealy advocates for advanced diagnostic testing to identify specific cancer markers and custom-tailor personal treatments accordingly. This can include genetic testing and assessments of cancer cell behavior.

Ty Bollinger Health Protocols

Here is a summary of Bollinger's cancer-fighting suggestions from his book *The Truth About Cancer*:

1. Dietary approaches

*Ketogenic Diet: Emphasizes high-fat, low-carbohydrate intake to potentially starve cancer cells of glucose.

*Plant-Based Diet: Advocates for a diet rich in fruits, vegetables, and whole grains to support overall health and potentially inhibit cancer growth.

*Juicing: Incorporates fresh vegetable and fruit juices to provide nutrients and support detoxification.

2. Supplementation

*Vitamin C therapy. High-dose intravenous vitamin C is discussed for its potential to kill cancer cells and support the immune system.

*Vitamin D. Supplementation for its role in immune function and potential anti-cancer effects.

*Curcumin. The active compound in turmeric is known for its anti-inflammatory and antioxidant properties.

3. Detoxification

*Coffee Enemas. Suggested for detoxifying the liver and aiding in the removal of toxins.

*Colon Cleanses. Focus on clearing the digestive tract to improve overall health.

5. Exercise. Regular physical activity is encouraged to enhance overall well-being and support immune function.

6. Stress reduction. Techniques such as meditation, yoga, and deep breathing to reduce stress and support healing.

7. Alternative therapies

*Ozone Therapy. Utilizes ozone to increase oxygen levels in the body and potentially target cancer cells.

*Hyperbaric oxygen therapy. Involves breathing pure oxygen in a pressurized room to improve oxygen delivery to tissues and support healing.

8. Herbal and natural remedies

*Essiac tea. An herbal formula claimed to have cancer-fighting properties.

*Graviola (Soursop). A plant with encouraging anti-cancer effects.

9. Visualization and meditation. Presents techniques to support mental and emotional well-being, which may contribute to overall health.

10. Traditional Chinese Medicine (TCM). This approach uses acupuncture, herbal remedies, and other practices to support cancer treatment and recovery.

11. Boost the body's immune response to better fight cancer. Ultimately, the body heals itself of cancer.

Another therapy of interest discussed in Bollinger's *The Truth About Cancer* is the use of cannabis, specifically its THC and CBD elements. Bollinger discusses the use of high-THC oil and high-CBD oil as part of a cancer treatment regimen. He emphasizes the potential benefits of using these cannabis formulations for their anti-cancer properties, particularly for their ability to induce apoptosis in cancer cells and reduce tumor growth. The specific formulations include Rick

Simpson Oil (RSO), a highly concentrated THC oil, and CBD-rich oils, known for their anti-inflammatory and tumor-reducing effects.

Here are three studies that have shown positive results in using cannabis for cancer treatment:

Guzmán, M. (2003). "Cannabinoids: potential anticancer agents." *Nature Reviews Cancer*, 3(10), 745-755. Demonstrated that cannabinoids, notably THC, can induce apoptosis (programmed cell death) in glioma cells and inhibit tumor growth in animal models.

Velasco, G., et al. (2004). "Cannabinoids and gliomas." *Molecular Neurobiology*, 29(2), 97-106. Found that cannabinoids selectively target and kill malignant glioma cells without affecting normal brain cells.

Russo, E., & Guy, G. W. (2006). "A tale of two cannabinoids: The therapeutic rationale for combining tetrahydrocannabinol and cannabidiol." *Medical Hypotheses*, 66(2), 234-246. Showed the synergistic effects of THC and CBD in treating cancer, suggesting enhanced efficacy in reducing tumor growth when used together.

A Friend Who Healed Her Father of Cancer

As an adjunct to Bollinger's suggestion and the cited studies above addressing cannabis as a possible cancer treatment, I am sharing an intriguing message I received. The following is part of a verbatim note from a woman who participated in a health & longevity Meetup group I created in 2023:

"Hi Michael,

I wanted to forward you the information on Cannabis. I hope you find this information useful and perhaps you can pass it on as you feel it may be helpful to others. Know that we are just passing on information that could be helpful like a supplement. Each person should consult their physician prior to trying out new avenues to health as we are not physicians and so each person that has this information must try at their own discretion and risk.

This is a formulation I used for my dad. These are the more formal formulation instructions that were supposed to help w/my dad and anyone else you know with the ailments outlined. Or, as we spoke about, anyone with a propensity to contract cancer/ tumors or have an autoimmune ailment . . . in the future which is probably the human population at large . . . due to all the toxins we put in the world! I know it stops seizures in Shiatzus (dogs) and Staffordshire terriers and eliminated lung cancer in my dad:-)"

Cannabis oil can be used for many purposes. I have two favorite purposes: for epilepsy and cancer. Cannabis cuts off the blood supply to cancer cells. There is not enough data currently available to thoroughly understand the benefits of all of the component cannabinoids as well as terpenes in cannabis. However, I have personal experience and circumstantial evidence that cannabis cures lung cancer. My dad had lung cancer, and I created the following oil extract, and his lung cancer went away.

Because of the inconsistency of my formulation and lack of data, I can only provide guidelines for what may help you and or your friends who are experiencing issues with cancer or other auto-immune (AI) illnesses such as epilepsy, Crohn's, diabetes, and Parkinson's and Cushing's Syndrome."

The sender then gave me her healing formula and prep instructions she claimed cured her father of lung cancer. Two of the web links she sent me to help me understand the cannabis ingredients were from Leafly.com. Of course, you are invited to explore cannabis treatment possibilities on such sites.

Gerson Cancer Therapy Protocols

Based on the research of Dr. Max Gerson and updated by his daughter Charlotte Gerson in her 2005 book *Healing the Gerson Way: Defeating Cancer and Other Chronic Diseases*, here is a summary of Gerson Therapy for fighting cancer:

1. Organic vegetarian diet. Consume a strict organic, plant-based diet high in potassium and low in sodium. Eliminate table salt from your diet. This diet is designed to provide the body with abundant nutrients, enzymes, and antioxidants.

2. Fresh organic juices. Drink up to 13 glasses of freshly made organic fruit and vegetable juices daily. These juices are consumed every hour and are believed to flood the body with essential nutrients while detoxifying the body.

3. Coffee enemas. Administer up to 5 coffee enemas per day for detoxification. The goal is stimulating the liver to release toxins and support the body's detoxification processes.

4. Nutritional supplements. Take specific vitamins, minerals, and enzymes, including:
*Potassium
*Lugol's Solution (potassium iodide, iodine, and water)
*Coenzyme Q10 injected with vitamin B12
*Vitamins A, C, and B3 (niacin)
*Flaxseed oil
*Pancreatic enzymes
*Pepsin (a stomach enzyme)

5. Food preparation. Prepare meals without salt, spices, or oils, and avoid aluminum and Teflon cookware or utensils.

6. Detoxification. Focus on removing toxins from the body through diet and organic coffee enemas. Also, consume castor oil and avoid toxic substances in processed foods, artificial additives, and non-organic produce.

7. Thyroid support. The therapy includes steps to support thyroid function, crucial for regulating metabolism and detoxification processes.

8. Rest and stress reduction. The Gerson Therapy emphasizes the importance of adequate rest, relaxation, and stress management, essential for healing.

9. Monitoring and personalization. Patients are closely monitored, and the therapy is personalized based on individual needs, with adjustments made as necessary to optimize results.

10. Extended therapy duration. Follow the Gerson Therapy for a minimum of 2 years.

It's important to note that while these are the protocols suggested by Gerson Therapy, always consult with qualified medical professionals before considering alternative cancer treatments.

The Gerson Therapy Coffee Enema Summary

Ingredients: 3 tablespoons of organic coffee, medium or dark roast to make 4 cups (1 liter) using distilled or filtered water.

*Boil 4 cups of distilled or filtered water in a pot.

*Add 3 tablespoons of organic coffee to the boiling water.

*Lower the heat and let the coffee simmer for 10-15 minutes.

*After simmering, remove the pot from heat and allow the coffee to cool to body temperature (98-104°F or 37-40°C).

*Strain the coffee using a fine mesh strainer or cheesecloth to remove all coffee grounds.

*Pour the cooled, strained coffee into an enema bag or pitcher.

*Lubricate the enema tip with a natural lubricant such as coconut oil.

*Lie on your **right** side with your knees drawn up, and gently insert the enema tip into the rectum.

*Allow the coffee to flow into the colon slowly.

*Try to retain the enema for 12-15 minutes before expelling.

Frequency. In Gerson Therapy, coffee enemas may be recommended several times daily, depending on the individual's health condition.

Potential benefits of coffee enemas:
*Stimulate bile production and liver detoxification.
*Enhance the removal of toxins and waste products from the body.
*Provide relief from pain and discomfort associated with body detoxification.

Dave Asprey Cancer-Fighting Recommendations

The biohacker and author of *Super Human* makes a case for the importance of Natural Killer (NK) cells, a type of lymphocyte, a vital immune system component. They play a crucial role in the body's defense against tumors and viral infections. Here's an overview of their characteristics, functions, and significance:
*NK cells originate from the bone marrow and are part of the innate immune system. They typically comprise about 5-15% of the circulating lymphocytes in the blood.
*NK cells express specific surface proteins, including CD56 and CD16, which help differentiate them from other lymphocytes, like T cells.
*NK cells can directly kill infected or cancerous cells by releasing cytotoxic granules containing perforin and granzymes, which induce apoptosis (programmed cell death).

Functions of Natural Killer Cells

*NK cells are particularly effective against viral infections. They can recognize and eliminate cells infected with viruses, often before the adaptive immune response is activated.
*Can identify and destroy malignant cells, contributing to the body's natural tumor surveillance mechanisms.
*In addition to their cytotoxic abilities, NK cells produce various cytokines (such as interferon-gamma) that help regulate immune responses and enhance the activity of other immune cells.

*Can modulate immune responses, influencing the activities of other immune cells, such as dendritic cells and T cells.

Activation and Regulation

NK cells are activated by a combination of signals, including stress-induced ligands on target cells, cytokines (like IL-2 and IL-12), and interactions with other immune cells. They also have inhibitory receptors that recognize normal "self" cells, preventing them from attacking healthy tissues.

NK Clinical Possibilities for Cancer Treatment

1. Cancer Immunotherapy. NK cells are being explored as a therapeutic target in cancer treatment. Approaches include enhancing their activity or using genetically engineered NK cells to improve their effectiveness against tumors.
2. Understanding NK cell function can help in the development of treatments for viral infections and immune-related disorders.
3. NK cells play a role in organ graft rejection and tolerance, making them relevant in organ transplantation research.
4. Natural killer cells are essential players in the immune system, providing rapid responses to viral infections and cancerous cells. Their unique properties and potential therapeutic applications make them a significant focus of research in immunology and medicine.

NK Cell Enhancement Protocols

Supplements, vitamins, and therapies have been shown to promote the growth and strength of natural killer (NK) cells. Some to consider:
1. Vitamin C enhances the function of NK cells and boosts overall immune response. Studies suggest vitamin C can stimulate NK cell activity and promote their proliferation.

2. Vitamin D is linked to enhanced immune function, including the activity of NK cells. Some studies indicate vitamin D can increase NK cell cytotoxicity, particularly in older adults.

3. Zinc plays a crucial role in immune function and has been shown to enhance NK cell activity. Zinc supplementation has been associated with improved NK cell numbers and function, especially in those with deficiencies.

4. Beta-glucans are polysaccharides found in the cell walls of fungi, yeast, and grains that can stimulate the immune system. Beta-glucans have been shown to enhance NK cell activity and proliferation, making them a popular supplement for immune support.

5. Elderberry is known for its antiviral properties and may enhance immune function. Studies suggest elderberry extracts can increase NK cell activity, particularly during viral infections.

6. Curcumin (Turmeric) has anti-inflammatory and antioxidant properties that may support immune function. Studies indicate that curcumin can enhance NK cell activity and improve immune responses.

7. Probiotics. Gut health is closely linked to immune function, and probiotics can help maintain a healthy gut microbiome. Certain probiotic strains have been shown to enhance NK cell activity and overall immune response.

8. Regular exercise has been shown to improve immune function, including NK cell activity. Physical activity can stimulate the proliferation and activity of NK cells, contributing to overall health.

9. Adequate sleep is crucial for optimal immune function. Studies show sleep deprivation can negatively affect NK cell activity, while good sleep quality supports immune health.

10. Stress management. Chronic stress can suppress immune function. Techniques like meditation, yoga, and mindfulness can help reduce stress and improve immune responses, including NK cell activity.

Incorporating these vitamins, supplements, and lifestyle practices can help enhance NK cell growth and strength. As always, it's important to consult with a healthcare provider before starting any new supplements or therapies.

Dr. Tom Rogers' Intriguing Recommendations

In his YouTube video "Fenbendazole and Artemisinin," Rogers details the cancer research and results of repurposing fenbendazole --- an inexpensive dog de-wormer! --- and artemisinin, also known as sweet wormwood, which has been used in traditional Chinese medicine for centuries.

Artemisinin is primarily known for its use in treating malaria due to its potent anti-parasitic properties and has shown promise in fighting cancer. When consumed appropriately, fenbendazole and artemisinin show little to no side effects.

Fenbendazole acts on cancer cells in the following ways:

1. It inhibits cancer cell mitosis, cell division, and replication.

2. Induces apoptosis, programmed cancer cell death.

3. Sensitizes cancer cells to more easily being killed by radiation treatment

4. Reactivates the p53 gene, the body's most potent cancer suppressor

5. Starves cancer by inhibiting glucose uptake by the cancer cells

For details on dosing, see Rogers' YouTube video referenced above.

CancerChoices.org's 7 Healing Practices

1. Explore what matters now. This is a reflective practice emphasized by CancerChoices.org, guiding individuals through pivotal moments in their lives, particularly during a cancer journey. It involves identifying the core values and priorities that matter most at the present moment, which can help in making informed decisions about treatments and lifestyle changes. For instance, someone might prioritize quality of life and opt for complementary therapies alongside conventional treatments. Alternatively, others might choose aggressive treatments to extend life at all costs. The process is deeply personal, encouraging individuals to align their actions with their values, resulting in a more fulfilling and intentional approach to living with cancer.

2. Healthy diet. A good diet involves nourishing yourself with food that promotes health and resilience against cancer and its side effects. This practice includes adopting a plant-based, whole-food diet emphasizing vegetables, fruits, whole grains, nuts, seeds, and healthy fats while limiting processed foods, red meat, and sugary drinks. Benefits of eating well include improved treatment responses, reduced inflammation, lower risk of recurrence, and better quality of life.

This approach can help manage symptoms like fatigue, depression, and gastrointestinal issues. It is essential to tailor your diet to your medical conditions and consult with healthcare providers, especially if you are experiencing side effects that impact eating.

3. Move. Engaging in physical activity can reduce cancer risk, promote health after a diagnosis, and alleviate some side effects of treatment. Activities include walking, gardening, dancing, swimming, and yoga. Moderate to vigorous exercise, such as brisk walking or resistance training, is particularly beneficial. It's vital to find enjoyable activities to maintain motivation and ensure safety by following your doctor's advice and gradually increasing intensity. Staying hydrated and moving safely is crucial for maximizing the benefits of physical activity during and after cancer treatment.

4. Manage stress. Stress management is crucial for people with cancer as it can directly impact health and recovery. Chronic stress can elevate hormone levels such as cortisol and adrenaline, which may suppress the immune system and promote inflammation. Techniques to manage stress include mindfulness practices like meditation and yoga, physical activities like tai chi and qigong, spending time in nature, and engaging in enjoyable activities. Additionally, ensuring sound sleep, seeking social support, and possibly using medication or herbal remedies can also help. The goal is to reduce overall stress and develop coping strategies for unavoidable stresses, ultimately creating a more favorable environment for healing and reducing the risk of cancer progression.

5. Quality sleep. Sleep is crucial for improving quality of life, managing cancer symptoms and side effects, and potentially enhancing treatment response. Sleep disruption is common in cancer patients due to stress, anxiety, and treatment side effects. Getting at least seven hours of sleep regularly is recommended to improve resilience and well-being. Adequate sleep helps reduce treatment side effects, cancer symptoms, and risk of recurrence. Disrupted sleep is linked to worse outcomes, whereas better sleep quality is associated with improved survival rates in advanced cancer patients. CancerChoices.org suggests addressing sleep issues by establishing a consistent sleep schedule and seeking medical advice if excessive sleepiness or insomnia persists. Integrating good sleep practices as part of an individualized plan can contribute to a less supportive environment for cancer development and progression.

6. Create a healing environment. This involves several key practices to enhance physical and emotional well-being, particularly for cancer patients. It includes establishing a personal sanctuary, a safe and calming space in one's home. Adjustments should be made to living spaces to ensure safety, especially if the individual is experiencing side effects from treatments. Increasing beneficial exposures to nature and daylight while minimizing harmful exposures to toxins, pollutants, and radiation is also critical. These practices collectively create an environment that supports healing by fostering physical safety, emotional calm, and a connection to nature.

7. Share love and support. This practice involves participating in supportive partnerships and communities, which can significantly benefit cancer patients. It encompasses forming a network of family, friends, neighbors, and community members to provide psychological, physical, and, if needed, financial help. This social support has been shown to improve survival rates, reduce cancer risk, alleviate treatment side effects, and enhance the overall quality of life. Recommendations include engaging in support groups, retreats, and online discussion forums to maintain social connections and reduce feelings of isolation.

From the menu items available on the ***CancerChoices.org*** homepage, select "Reviews of Complementary Therapies." Complementary cancer therapies are those used in addition to conventional treatments, such as chemotherapy, radiation, or surgery. For each complementary therapy, the website team searched for published medical studies confirm the following four medical benefits:

1. Improved treatment outcomes. Does the therapy improve survival, reduce metastases, shrink tumors, or reduce tumor markers? Does it enhance other treatments?

2. Optimization of your body terrain. Does the therapy address factors known to support the growth or spread of cancer?

3. Managing side effects and promoting wellness. Does the therapy prevent or reduce any of the common side effects of cancer treatments or symptoms of cancer?

4. Risk reduction. Does the therapy reduce the risks of cancer or its recurrence?

The team assesses whether study results are clinically relevant, the size of effects, and whether studies involve humans or only cells or animals. We evaluate whether studies are designed well enough to draw meaningful conclusions. We determine whether findings across studies are consistent or conflicting. We summarize and interpret each set of findings for you but also allow you to see details and sources if that interests you.

Therapies are rated on a 0–5-point scale to assess how strong the evidence is regarding questions that most people with cancer want to know:

1. Does this therapy improve treatment outcomes?

2. Does it improve my general health, resilience, and my body terrain? Does the therapy address these factors and others known to support the growth or spread of cancer when out of balance?

3. Potential side effects of some therapies may be bleeding and coagulation imbalance, body weight, high blood sugar and insulin resistance, hormone imbalance, immune function, inflammation, oxidative stress, and microbiome harm. Does the therapy manage potential side effects and symptoms?

4. Does the therapy reduce my risk of cancer or recurrence?

5. How do experts use this therapy?

6. What safety concerns do I need to know about?

7. What does it cost, and where can I find it?

I selected / high-graded the CancerChoices.org recommended therapies that show the highest positive ratings --- a rating of 4 or 5 --- on at least one of the Big Three questions from the 7 therapy rating questions above. My Big Three Questions of particular interest are Questions 1, 2, and 4 above: enhanced cancer treatment outcomes, improved general health & resilience, and reduced cancer risk or recurrence.

Here are my high-grade selections where a recommended cancer-fighting protocol receives at least one rating of 4 or 5 from CancerChoices.org:

***A Mediterranean diet** high in vegetables, fruits, whole grains, and olive oil and low in meat, sweets, and saturated fat. It is linked to lower risks of cancer and relief of some symptoms and imbalances common among people with cancer Ratings by CancerChoices.org on my Big Three Questions: 1, **4, 4**

***Calorie restriction and fasting**, whether for 12 or more hours every night or occasionally for more extended periods, can contribute to lower body weight, blood sugar, and insulin resistance, plus fewer unpleasant chemotherapy-related side effects. Ratings by CancerChoices.org on my Big Three Questions: 2,**5**,3

***Berberine**, an active ingredient in several plants, shows positive effects in managing high blood sugar and excess body weight, plus a lower risk of colorectal cancer. Ratings by CancerChoices.org on my Big Three Questions: 1,**4**,3

***Green tea and its extracts** may provide substantial benefits for body terrain factors, especially body weight, high blood sugar and insulin resistance, inflammation, and oxidative stress, which are linked to cancer development and growth. Ratings by CancerChoices.org on my Three Questions: 2,**4**,4

***Quercetin**, found in many plant-based foods and available as a supplement, is linked to better body terrain and significantly lower inflammation. Quercetin is available as a supplement. Ratings by CancerChoices.org on my Big Three Questions: 1,**5**,3

***Resveratrol** is a polyphenol that can reduce oxidative stress. Resveratrol is found in grape skins and seeds, peanuts, blueberries, cranberries, and cocoa but is usually taken as a supplement. Supplements are generally low-cost and widely available. Ratings by CancerChoices.org on my Big Three Questions: 2,**4**,2

***Vitamin D** is a hormone created by the body by exposure to ultraviolet B (UVB) from the sun. It can also be taken as a supplement in either soft gel or liquid form and is found naturally in some foods. Ratings by CancerChoices.org on my Big Three Questions: **5,5,5**

***Grapes and products made from grapes** may promote body terrain factors known to be important in cancer, including better blood sugar and insulin levels and less oxidative stress. Ratings by CancerChoices.org on my Big Three Questions: 0,**4**,2

***Melatonin**, a hormone produced by the pineal gland in your brain, helps regulate your sleep and wake cycles. Minimal amounts of melatonin are found in fruits, nuts, olive oil, and wine. Available as a supplement and as a sleep aid. Ratings by CancerChoices.org on my Big Three Questions: **5,4,4**

***Probiotics** are living microorganisms that provide a health benefit, and prebiotics are fibers that feed these friendly bacteria, primarily in your gut. These therapies, found in certain foods or as supplements, can manage gastrointestinal symptoms and body terrain factors common in cancer, and they may lead to better recovery from surgery. Ratings by CancerChoices.org on my Big Three Questions: 3.**5,4**

***Reishi** mushrooms have medicinal properties and are available in dried form and as a supplement in capsules. It is used in cancer care to enhance chemo/radiotherapy treatment. Ratings by CancerChoices.org on my Big Three: 3,4,2

***Vitamin C** is an essential nutrient for growth, development, and healing. Vitamin C deficiency is linked to an increased risk of several diseases, including cancer. Ratings by CancerChoices.org on my Big Three Questions: 3,**4**,4

***Hyperthermia** is a type of treatment in which tumors or body tissues are heated as high as 113°F (45°C) to damage or kill cancer cells, sometimes with little or no harm to normal tissue. Ratings by CancerChoices.org on my Big Three Questions: 4,2,3

***Non-aspirin nonsteroidal anti-inflammatory drugs (NSAIDs)**, including non-prescription ibuprofen and naproxen, are used to reduce inflammation. Ratings by CancerChoices.org on my Big Three Questions: **4,5,5**

***Aspirin** is widely available as an over-the-counter medication used to reduce inflammation and related pain. General use became widespread before its safety was fully assessed. The use of aspirin presents more risks than many people are aware of. Ratings by CancerChoices.org on my Big Three Questions: **5,5,5**

***Metformin** is a prescription drug used to control high blood glucose in type 2 diabetes. Some integrative cancer care physicians use metformin off-label for cancer treatment, use that has not yet received FDA approval. Every US state allows drugs to be used off-label as long as enough evidence supports its use. Ratings by CancerChoices.org on my Big Three Questions: 3,**5**,3

Best of the Best Recommendations

When I high-grade the Best of the Best recommended therapies suggested by CancerChoices.org, here are the clear-cut winners:
*Aspirin (5,5,5),
*Vitamin D (5,5,5),
*Non-aspirin nonsteroidal anti-inflammatory drugs (NSAIDs), including ibuprofen and naproxen (4,5,5)
*Melatonin (5,4,4)

These four make the elite All-Star Team, all readily available, inexpensive, over-the-counter products. Of course, if you choose to incorporate these into your daily health and cancer-fighting regimen, do your research and consult with a qualified medical or nutritional specialist. Learn the dosing, the frequency, and the potential side effects.

CancerChoices.org Mission Review

CancerChoices.org is a fantastic, comprehensive resource for information on cancer treatment and complementary therapies. The website focuses on providing **evidence-based**, patient-centered information to help people make informed decisions about their cancer care. Here's a summary of what CancerChoices.org --- **a 5-Star resource** --- offers you and its approach to cancer treatment possibilities:

1. Evidence-Based Information
***Comprehensive reviews.** CancerChoices.org provides detailed reviews of various cancer treatments, including

conventional, integrative, and complementary options. The reviews are based on scientific evidence and aim to present an objective overview of each treatment's efficacy, safety, and potential benefits.

***Current research.** The site offers updates on recent research and clinical trials, helping users stay informed about the latest developments in cancer treatment.

2. Integrative and Complementary Therapies

***Holistic approach.** The website emphasizes integrative cancer care, which combines conventional treatments (such as chemotherapy, radiation, and surgery) with complementary therapies (such as nutrition, mind-body practices, and herbal supplements).

***Complementary therapies.** Information is provided on various complementary therapies, including acupuncture, massage therapy, nutritional support, and stress reduction techniques, with a focus on how these can be used alongside conventional treatments to improve quality of life.

3. Patient-Centered Resources

***Personal stories**. CancerChoices.org features personal stories and testimonials from individuals who have explored different treatment options, offering insights into their experiences and outcomes.

***Decision-making tools**. The site includes tools and resources to help patients and their families make informed decisions about their treatment options, including questions to ask healthcare providers and guidance on evaluating treatment choices.

4. Professional Contributions

***Expert opinions.** The site includes contributions from various experts in the fields of oncology, integrative medicine, and complementary therapies. These contributions provide authoritative perspectives on different treatments.

***Collaborative approach.** CancerChoices.org often collaborates with healthcare professionals to ensure the accuracy and reliability of the information presented.

5. Educational Resources. The website offers educational guides, articles, and other resources to help users understand different aspects of cancer care, including treatment options, side effects management, and strategies for maintaining overall health.

6. Focus on Personalization. Individualized Care: CancerChoices.org emphasizes the importance of personalized cancer care plans tailored to each patient's unique needs and preferences. It encourages patients to work closely with their healthcare team to develop a treatment plan that aligns with their individual goals and circumstances.

7. Advocacy and Support. Supportive Community: The site provides information on support groups, advocacy organizations, and other resources that can assist patients and their families throughout their cancer journey.

CancerChoices.org is dedicated to helping individuals explore a wide range of treatment possibilities, focusing on integrating conventional and complementary approaches to provide comprehensive, patient-centered care.

Step 7 – Write Out a Step-by-Step Winning Battle Plan

Once you have your hope, your will, and your commitment and have begun your comprehensive research, it's time to begin to crystallize your written Master Battle Plan. Adopting the attitude and tactics of a warrior is appropriate.

Often, adopting strategies, therapies, and treatments for optimal health involves many battles in an ongoing war. A war against our lazy selves, misinformation, lack of knowledge and investigative research, accepted ideas of "normal," and a sad resignation to "that's just how it is."

Doctors and medical "experts" do not have all the answers that may be available for you seeking healing from your cancer. Doctors and experts may help you, but no one cares about your health or your loved one as much as you.

So, I invite you to assume a military strategist's mindset to fight every day to ensure optimal health, enabling you to actively live, love, and laugh well beyond projected life expectancies. Toward this end, the ancient Chinese book *The Art of War* provides some inspirational strategies and tactics.

A Quick Strategic Overview of Successfully Prosecuting War

Written sometime between the 5th and 3rd centuries BC, *The Art of War* is a battlefield treatise attributed to Chinese military leader Sun Tsu. The book offers timeless principles on warfare, strategies, tactics, and leadership in conducting a war, with obvious applications to everyday life. Tsu advocates cunning over force and victory without doing battle.

To be successful, you, the general, must know both your own and your enemy's strengths, weaknesses, and vulnerabilities. Deception, adaptability, and maneuvering strategically are key. Exploit your enemy's weaknesses, strike swiftly, and secure resources. Protect your supply lines, fortify your position, and choose advantageous terrain. Motivate your troops, reward success, and punish failures. Be calm and adaptable to situations, like water flowing around obstacles and through changing terrain, remaining resolute to winning. Victory comes from calculated moves, not brute force. Tenacious dedication and discipline are essential.

Endorsements and High Praise for the book The Art of War

*Famous American World War II General George S. Patton: "In reading *The Art of War* by Sun Tzu, I was struck by the fact that the principles of war he lays down are exactly the same as those I have learned by long experience."

*Napoleon Bonaparte, French Emperor and renowned European military leader: "*The Art of War* is Napoleon's Bible."

*Confederate Civil War General Stonewall Jackson: "I find in Sun Tzu a book of real practical philosophy. Here are condensed the results of long experience and profound reflection. It is the work of a great mind."

*Supreme Allied Commander in World War II and US President Dwight Eisenhower: "I still read Sun Tzu. His writings are full of wisdom. His name belongs on the short list of the great military leaders of history."

Cancer-Fighting Applications of Sun Tsu's Ideas

The Art of War is not just a military treatise; it offers valuable insights applicable to various aspects of life, from business and politics to personal interactions and self-improvement. By understanding and applying these timeless principles, you can gain valuable strategic thinking skills and navigate challenging situations with wisdom and foresight, including applying Tsu's wisdom to your health and cancer-fighting game plan.

Here, as in my book *Optimal Health and Longevity: Adopting Battle Tactics from Sun Tsu's The Art of War Volume 1* (available at MichaelGormanBooks.com), I apply Sun Tsu's wise tactics and strategies to maximizing your health --- physical, mental, emotional, and spiritual --- and, hopefully, extending your active time on this Earth by years. Perhaps many, many years, General.

Defeat What Seems Impossible

Sun Tsu: "Victory comes from finding opportunities in the impossible."

Don't give up on seemingly impossible health goals. Seek alternative solutions, consult experts, and believe in your potential for growth. See challenges as opportunities for learning and improvement. Never stop looking for ways to extend your healthy lifespan.

*Reframe challenges as opportunities. Instead of viewing setbacks as failures, analyze them as learning experiences.

*View obstacles as opportunities to discover new solutions, build resilience, and strengthen your commitment.

*Embrace non-traditional exercise activities. Instead of clinging to conventional cancer treatments, explore the myriads of successful alternative healing possibilities. New therapies, drugs, supplements, and effective lifestyle tweaks are being discovered constantly.

*Challenge beliefs that limit you. Instead of accepting "I can't" as your answer, reframe negative self-talk. Break down seemingly impossible goals into achievable steps and witness your potential for growth. "I can, and I will."

*Leverage tech and useful resources. Instead of feeling isolated on your health journey, join online communities, utilize health apps, or consult remote health professionals. Connect with others and access resources beyond your immediate environment. Meetup (Meetup.com) cancer support groups offer great options. If no such group exists in your location, consider creating the group yourself.

Considerations for Building Your Master Battle Plan

I suggest that a legal pad and pen be your constant companions. So they are not forgotten, write down ideas and updates as they come to you without having to start your laptop or open your cell phone.

In the Immediate

If you or a loved one have Stage 4 cancer, immediate action is necessary. Every hour is critical. YOU must act now! There is hope beyond what your doctor may offer in the form of simple, noninvasive, low to no side effects therapies to implement this moment. Now, not tomorrow.

As I write this portion of the book, I am thinking back to the tragic situation of the cancer-stricken 52-year-old woman whose doctors and family did NOTHING to help her in her last month of life in July/August 2024. All parties had nothing to lose by trying alternative non-invasive therapies with minimal or no side effects that may have helped her. Sadly, and infuriating for me, we will never know. The passive family deferred to her doctor as God, a god who did nothing but pronounce a death sentence.

In crafting a battle plan, you, the warrior cancer patient or loving advocate general, must consider IMMEDIATE non-invasive, cancer-fighting actions, most of which have minimal or no side effects with reasonable, effective doses. ALWAYS do your research. When in doubt, consult multiple holistic medical professionals.

Immediate non-invasive therapies

1. Adequate hydration with clean, purified water
2. Cancer-fighting and immune-enhancing, non-toxic, organic foods
3. Avoidance of cancer-feeding processed foods and sugar
4. Limit the use of antibiotics
5. Ensure quality sleep
6. Liposomal Vitamin C (If unable to eat or swallow, research intravenous dosing of Vitamin C.)
7. Vitamin D + Vitamin K.
8. Other cancer-fighting vitamins and supplements, such as Curcumin, CoQ10, Green Tea Extract, Omega-3 Fatty Acids, NAC, Resveratrol, Selenium, Melatonin, and Magnesium.

9. Ibuprofen, naproxen, and aspirin. Research effective and reasonable doses and durations for each.
10. Off-label compounds such as ivermectin, fenbendazole, and artemisinin.
11. Stress relief techniques, including overcoming fear
12. Deep breathing
13. Reaffirming a passionate reason to live
14. Removal of environmental toxins --- pesticides, herbicides, asbestos, radon, toxic mold
15. Active involvement with a caring social network and family
16. Hyperbaric Oxygen Therapy
17. Sauna therapy. Even hot, steamy showers can have healing benefits.

Your Comprehensive Master Battle Plan Creation

For your cancer's ultimate defeat, be guided by the following questions or suggestions as you write out The Plan:
1. Assert and remind yourself at all times that YOU are in charge of your health and decisions that affect your cancer treatment. Your doctor is not God.
2. Your Master Battle Plan must be *written* so it may be reviewed daily, present you with important reminders, and changes and updates recorded. You cannot possibly remember all that must be done to stop your cancer and prevent its recurrence or another disease.
3. Seek out holistic or naturopathic medical professionals for consultation and potential treatments for your cancer.
4. Always get a second opinion. Maybe three and four.
5. What type and stage of cancer are you dealing with?
6. What may have caused your cancer? This could prevent the worsening of your disease and eliminate its future recurrence.
7. What are the available treatment options and their potential side effects? For starters, refer to the recommendations of the

Cancer Research All-Star Team highlighted earlier in this book.

8. What are the goals of the treatment, e.g., cure, control, or merely symptom relief?

9. How will treatments impact the quality of your day-to-day life? Prepare. Adapt.

10. Are surgery, chemotherapy, or radiation treatments really the right course at this time?

11. Can surgery, chemotherapy, or radiation actually worsen my condition? You must know the potential downside effects of all these. For instance, chemotherapy can knock out your immune system, and radiation may kill healthy cells and tissues.

12. Today, determine what proven healing treatments and therapies you can personally implement right now, immediately, such as diet, movement, and sleep, as supported by your comprehensive research. See pages 8 or 114 to review research-supported measures you can implement immediately to fight your cancer. For example, staying hydrated with purified water, taking liposomal Vitamin C, making changes to ensure quality sleep, implementing stress relief measures, dedicating regular walking and exercise time, avoiding processed foods and sugar, and eating quality organic superfoods are a few obvious do-it-yourself healing steps. Start now, today. Write these into your Master Battle Plan.

13. What long-term, proven lifestyle changes --- life purpose, diet, exercise, social support, stress management --- should be implemented to support the doctor-recommended treatment plan and your own plan to promote healing?

14. The first line of your body's defense against disease or the recurrence of disease is your immune system. A healthy immune system positively supports and enhances the effectiveness of all cancer treatments and therapies you may choose. You must rebuild a damaged immune system and maintain its health.

15. What are common thread healing and preventative approaches recommended by cancer survivors and skilled and effective cancer specialists and researchers?
16. Are there clinical trials or new treatment options that you should consider?
17. What resources and support systems --- medical teams, mental health support groups, mental health professionals, websites, cancer survivor groups --- are available?
18. What are the expected timelines for treatment and recovery?
19. How and by whom will the progress of the treatment be monitored and evaluated? How will you ensure timely test and evaluation results? Anticipate delays and push to prevent them.
20. What follow-up care and screening tests will be necessary or optional after treatment ends?
21. What is the plan for managing and mitigating side effects and complications of the treatment(s)?
22. What is the likelihood of cancer recurrence, and what steps can you take to reduce this risk? Write these.
23. What symptoms should you watch for that could indicate a recurrence or new cancer?
24. Research relentlessly and beware of false information and the many cancer scams meant to victimize the fearful and vulnerable.
25. How will the financial aspects of treatment be managed (insurance, out-of-pocket costs, assistance programs)? Bottom line consideration: Are you willing to put a dollar limit on your health? Remember, there is no evidence that you can take it with you.
26. For the love of yourself and someone you advocate for, vow every day to do the necessary work every day. Write about how you will do this in your Master Battle Plan.
27. Update and tweak your written Master Battle Plan on a regular basis.

Step 8 – Take Action! Implement Your Battle Plan

Your commitment and your *written* battle plan are now in place. The enemy, the roadblocks, and potential challenges have been identified. Adjustments and maneuvers will be required, but you are ready. Brief your team, even if it's just you today, and plan to attack and take that distant hill. It's time to go to war. At least one important life is at stake.

I emphasize a *written* Battle Plan because there is too much necessary information that must be laid out, organized, prioritized, remembered, and constantly referred to. It is impossible to do all this in your head. Write your plan on your PC or a legal pad. Add ideas, delete the necessary, and continuously fine-tune. Laziness or carelessness are not options when your life is at stake.

Refer to and begin marking off action items on your to-do list: research, reading, YouTube, cancer support websites, emails, phone calls, etc. Expect challenges and embrace them. Welcome your opportunities for courage, determination, and resourcefulness.

Step 9 --- Use Regular Testing and Measurements to Know Your Progress and Effectiveness of Your Master Battle Plan

Tests and measurements are used to detect cancer, monitor treatment effectiveness, and prevent it. These tests will help clarify the status of your cancer, suggest appropriate therapies and treatments, and measure your healing progress.

Here are numerous valuable tools:

1. Biomarker testing. These search for genes, proteins, and other substances that can provide information about a specific cancer. The test can guide treatment selection, especially for targeted therapies and immunotherapies. It may involve testing tumor tissue or blood samples. Examples include PSA for prostate cancer and BCR-ABL for chronic myeloid leukemia

2. Imaging tests. X-rays, CT scans, MRIs, and PET scans can reveal the location and size of tumors. Used for initial diagnosis and to monitor treatment response

3. Blood tests. These check for levels of substances released by cancer cells or affected organs. Can indicate tumor growth or shrinkage

4. Tumor marker tests. Measure specific proteins or other molecules released by tumors. Used to monitor cancer progression and treatment effectiveness

5. Physical exams and symptom assessment. Regular check-ups to look for any changes or new symptoms

6. Functional assessments. Measures of physical function like the ECOG scale or Karnofsky Performance Status (KPS). Can indicate how cancer/treatment is impacting daily activities. The KPS evaluates a patient's functional status and ability to perform daily activities to help determine if patients can receive chemotherapy, if dose adjustments are needed, and to assess the cancer prognosis. Scores range from 0 to 100, the latter being perfect health. So, the higher the score, the better the prognosis.

7. Quality of life assessments. Questionnaires like FACT-G are used to evaluate overall well-being and function.

8. Genetic testing. These can discover inherited cancer risk genes to then create preventative measures.

Tests used for prevention and early detection:

9. Standard cancer screening tests. Mammograms, colonoscopies, Pap tests, and others for detecting cancer early in high-risk or general populations. *Research test risks.*

10. The Galleri Test, created by the Grail Corporation, is an early-detection blood test that screens for 50 different cancers before symptoms are evident. I have completed this test.
11. Lifestyle assessments. Evaluations are made of your diet, physical activity, and tobacco/alcohol use to identify modifiable risk factors. Recommendations are then given.

The specific tests used depend on the type of cancer, stage, and individual patient factors. Regular monitoring with a combination of these methods helps guide treatment decisions and assess effectiveness. As an educated Health Warrior, assertively lobby to have these tests performed in light of your condition and health goals.

Step 10 --- Adjust and Fine-Tune Your Master Battle Plan

Depending on the direction and progress of your healing, your growing research knowledge, new challenges or obstacles, and your health victories or failures, your Master Battle Plan will require adjustments. In a worst-case scenario, radical adjustments may be needed. Possibilities include finding a new doctor, insisting on alternative treatments and therapies you have diligently researched, ramping up your research, or traveling to and staying at a private cancer treatment center. Be assertive, fueled by knowledge, self-love, and your Noble Purpose.

If your healing and recovery are progressing positively, additional health and healing protocols may need to be added. For instance, add to or uptick your exercise regimen, continue cleaning up your diet, or dedicate time to ridding your yard and home of carcinogenic toxins.

Step 11 --- Reaffirm Your Commitment to Never Surrender

Every righteous war has daily challenges before final victory is achieved. Of course, the cancer war may be extended or never-ending. Still, individual battles can be won to promote and lengthen a happy, functional, active, and fulfilling life toward the Final Victory. Take heart.

"Believe you can, and you're halfway there." President Theodore Roosevelt

"It does not matter how slowly you go as long as you do not stop." Confucius

"If you can't fly, then run; if you can't run, then walk; if you can't walk, then crawl, but whatever you do, keep moving forward." MLK, Jr.

"Fall seven times; stand up eight." Japanese Proverb

You must remind yourself every day about the Why of actively continuing to fight on. Why do you or who you advocate for want --- need --- to live?

Ponder and recite aloud your Noble Purpose every day. The world and those you love and care about need what only you can offer: your love, your gifts, and your talents. Living your Noble Purpose can be as simple as time spent in conversation, attentive listening, and offering encouragement and suggestions born from experience. You can help others, including the clerk at Walmart, by making them feel good about themselves on their Life Journey. "Thank you. (Big smile) I really appreciate your help and hope the rest of your day rocks!"

For those living alone, consider a four-legged companion, Fido or Fluffy. Our furry companions depend on us. On a personal note, besides The World needing me every day, I know that my cats --- Squeaky, Sasha, and The Bub --- need me and the loving care, engaging interactions, and snacks I provide. My clowns are additional incentives for me to be healthy, active, and safe. Safe? Yup. If I am tempted to drive a little too fast on a winding country road to get home to my cat family, I remind myself to slow down because these special creatures need me healthy and alive.

Farther along the road of reasons for fighting with no thought of surrender, consider any promises you have made. "Honey, when you grow up and get married, I will dance at your wedding." "Sweetheart, when you graduate from college, we will take a trip around the world to celebrate, you and me." "I promise myself to build a cabin in the woods with my own hands."

A couple of promises I have made . . . In 1987, at the funeral of a classmate, I promised all my friends there that I will attend ALL of their memorials and speak of some fond memories with them. Also, I have promised two of my friends that I will take them fishing to celebrate their 100th birthdays in 2051. When I row them down the river on those days, I will be 101. I WILL make good on my promises, just like you should make good on yours.

If you have not made any promises to someone or yourself, do so. When you have fulfilled your promises, immediately make more. In doing so, you have more reasons to fight on. Make BIG promises you feel obligated to fulfill. Never reach the finish line.

Expect, Prepare For, and Embrace Challenges

As I slide behind the wheel of my 4Runner, I talk to myself. Often, out loud: "I expect and embrace any and all challenges from careless or rude drivers I will meet. I will not surrender my emotions and mental health to anyone. I will respond with love and courtesy to my fellow travelers who have their own Life Journey. As best I can, I wish them well. These will be opportunities for calm, patience, and character growth. Bring it on!"

As mentioned in Step 2 of formulating your effective

cancer-fighting game plan, one of the challenges we all must face daily is our inclination toward laziness, a condition built into our human nature. Previously, I have made references to M. Scott Peck's 1978 book *The Road Less Traveled*, a work I have read no less than four times.

You may recall that Peck pointed to the challenge of laziness in recounting his interactions with many hundreds of mental health patients he dealt with over decades. Many of his patients struggled for months or years to understand, with his therapeutic help, what their psychological and/or emotional roadblocks were to experiencing fuller, happier, and controlled lives. Once the necessary insights and understanding of the problems were discovered, a game plan was formulated to heal the patient. It was, of course, incumbent on the patient to implement, to work, the healing process. Peck observed that many would not do the work or the follow-up necessary to finally defeat their challenges. Peck contends this is due to their --- and our --- innate laziness.

Laziness is the well-trodden Path of Least Resistance. It is always easiest to do nothing, requiring no energy, thought, discipline, or work.

Laziness May Incline You to Say, "My doctor is God! I will obey"

In November 2024, I continued to get sad updates about the husband who lost his wife in her battle against cancer, which pushed me to write this book. The family deferred to the woman's doctor in all decisions, including no helpful therapies and no simple, noninvasive nothing-to-lose alternative approaches, allowing the woman to suffer and die. Today, I heard that the distraught husband is planning a lawsuit.

Your "path of least resistance" may be to stand down and obey your doctor. Don't do it. You must be the proactive general willing to do the work. Recognizing our inclination toward laziness can somewhat blunt its power. Identify and defeat the innate enemy, your laziness, to effectively prosecute your war against cancer.

Avoid Time-Wasting Activities and Stay Organized

Time is precious. You must protect your time. There are many distractions and time-wasters that call to us from our TVs, cell phones, and personal computers. And, of course, there are legitimate projects and activities that summon us, such as household chores, shopping, exercise activities, and friends & family communications and events.

Dedicating some time at the start of each day to prioritize your activities and the organization of your day is imperative. Make this a habit. As a general prosecuting a war, this is a necessary strategy.

Writing out an activity to-do list every morning, I believe, is an unavoidable "must". The visual reminders and checking off of your completed activities are effective and impactful.

So, embrace the challenges, do the work --- because you MUST live your Noble Purpose and make good on your promises --- win each battle, and finally emerge victorious. Boldly pursue supportive cancer remedies with medical professionals. Know you will encounter frustrating delays and postponements. Keep pushing. Your health, maybe your life or that of someone you love is at stake. You can be courteous while at the same time demanding the necessary time and attention you require. Seek out other doctors who have the immediate time and treatments you need. Push the heavy ball up the hill. "No" or "Not now" are not acceptable answers to your critical needs.

Surrender is not an option, General.

MORE HEALING TOPICS OF INTEREST & REMINDERS

A Loving, Healing Companion by Your Side

Never underestimate the cancer-healing power of a pet. They will love you unconditionally, a never-ending source of joy and amusement.

In an October 2023 article entitled "Breast Cancer Treatment and Recovery: Pets' Roles as Emotional Buffers and Stressors" in *BMC Women's Health* talks about a study focused on breast cancer patients and showed that pets can serve as emotional buffers, improving mental health and quality of life during and after cancer treatment. Pets provide companionship and reduce loneliness, both crucial for coping with the psychological challenges of cancer recovery.

A meta-analysis of studies involving data from 3.8 million patients showed that dog owners experienced a 24% reduced risk in all-cause mortality, a 31% reduction in mortality due to cardiovascular issues, and a 65% reduced risk of mortality after a heart attack.

The Cornell University Feline Health Center cited various studies showing the benefits of interacting with cats. These interactions decrease stress levels by reducing cortisol (a hormone, too much of which can lead to weight gain, muscle weakness, anxiety, and depression) and increase positive feelings, thus contributing to both physical and psychological health.

Additionally, caring for a pet provides structure and routine to your day, which can be particularly beneficial for individuals struggling with depression, lack of direction, or purpose. Your loving companion cat, dog, or monkey needs you happy and healthy. They depend on you.

A Too-Often Overlooked Health Protocol for Defeating and Preventing Cancer: Adequate Hydration

It is not common in all my cancer research to find an emphasis on, or even mention, the importance of drinking adequate clean water.

The body, its tissues, and cells need nutrition and water. Water, not fruit juice, soda drinks, coffee, or whiskey. The human body is typically 50 – 60% water, depending on the degree of hydration.

Approximately 70% to 80% of a typical body cell is water. Sufficient water content is crucial for numerous cellular functions, including maintaining cell shape, enabling biochemical reactions, and facilitating the transport of nutrients and waste products.

More fun facts, examples of tissues and organs and their ideal water composition: your lungs are 83% water; muscles and kidneys, 79%; brain and heart, 73%; skin, 64%,, and bones, 31%.

Complications from dehydration include:

*Increased frequency of headaches

*Dizziness

*Fatigue

*Dry or flaky skin

*Constipation

*Difficulty swallowing

*Reduced muscle strength, power and endurance

*Mental status changes (impaired mood, concentration, attention and focus, reaction speed, short-term memory) and even delirium

*High blood pressure

*Kidney stones

*Decreased efficiency and effectiveness of immune system function

Preventing dehydration is vital to everyone, but especially

for people with cancer. Hydration is widely recommended in both conventional and complementary approaches to cancer care. By the time you feel thirsty, you are most likely dehydrated. Be proactive. I recommend setting the alarm on your cell phone to sound every hour: get up & move, drink water, and do some impact breathing.

Clean Your Water

Water can be toxic, contaminated with heavy metals, fluoride, and plastics. My research indicates that 73% of American municipal water supplies contain added fluoride, supposedly beneficial to oral health.

Here are three — there are more — studies citing the health hazards of fluoridated water. All agree that fluoride added to water supplies causes neurodevelopmental problems, especially in children, who exhibit significantly lower IQs as a result.

1. The Lancet Neurology (2014)
2. The Journal of American Medicine (2019)
3. Environmental Health Perspectives (2012)

While plastic bottles have revolutionized the convenience of purchasing and storing drinking water, contamination concerns exist. Here's a brief overview:

*Research indicates that tiny plastic particles, known as microplastics, may leach into water from plastic bottles. These particles can come from the bottle or the environment during the bottling process.

*Chemicals like bisphenol A (BPA) and phthalates, used in the production of plastic, can potentially leach into bottled water, especially when bottles are exposed to high temperatures or stored for long periods.

*Some studies have linked plastic-contaminated water to hormone disruption, increased oxidative stress, and other health concerns.

There's a simple home remedy: purify your water with a countertop distiller. I purchased a quality distiller on Amazon for about $250. I have a handheld water quality testing device to measure the change in purification from my tap water to my distilled water. The meter detects the dissolved impurities in the water before and after. My tap water registers a reading of "56", while my distilled water reads "0".

At no time in my distilling process does the water contact anything plastic. The receptacle pitcher which catches the water is made of glass. I store my water only in glass containers.

How much water is recommended should be typically consumed throughout the day to be healthily dehydrated? Take your body weight in pounds, divide this number by 2, and you arrive at the number of fluid ounces of water to drink. For example, 160 lbs. / 2 = 80 ounces of water per day.

You Are What You Eat --- Don't Feed Cancer

The Enticing Traps of the Common American Diet

We have been conditioned --- trained --- to love sugar and good-tasting processed foods. We can crave pastries, chips, soft drinks, ice cream, boxed breakfast cereals, pasta, bread, pizza, deep-fried or processed meats, and French fries. For some of us, kettle-cooked chips are heroin in a bag.

Cooking can be time-consuming work. Busy people seek convenience. Ready-to-eat or take & bake foods are fast and easy. Dining out is fun with family and friends.

Organic food, free of deadly pesticides and herbicides, is expensive.

Perhaps the #1 cancer-fighting protocol, confirmed by

ALL of the experts cited here and every survivor and researcher I have ever listened to, watched, or read, verifies that "you are what you eat." An unhealthy diet commonly leads to cancer.

In a November 2024 video interview on Rumble.com entitled "America's Food Is Poison," Johns Hopkins surgeon and *Blind Spots* author Dr. Marty Makary states, "Food is medicine . . . Maybe we need to talk about school lunch programs instead of giving every kid Ozempic (a drug used for blood glucose control and weight management) . . . And maybe we need to talk about the toxins, pesticides, and chemicals added to make food addictive. We can't just talk about chemotherapy for cancer without talking about its underlying causes. We didn't talk (in medical school) about the fact that 82% of research (independent) studies showed that many chemical food additives are harmful, while 93% of studies funded by the food industry showed that they were not bad for you. We can't keep going down this path of poisoning the food supply and just medicating everybody."

You, Health Warrior, need to forgo foods that are strictly determined by taste, convenience, and cost. Many common "foods" are poisonous. Summon your will and discipline to eat right. There can be no compromise. Your long, healthy life depends on it.

Deadly, Cancer-Causing Residues on Food

Pest and weed spray residue on foods will poison you, just as they are meant to kill weeds and insects.

Every year, the Environmental Working Group (EWG) releases its "Dirty Dozen" — a list of the 12 non-organic fruits and vegetables highest in pesticide contamination.

The 2024 EWG.org Dirty Dozen:
1. Strawberries
2. Spinach
3. Kale, collard & mustard greens
4. Grapes
5. Peaches
6. Pears
7. Nectarines
8. Apples
9. Bell and hot peppers
10. Cherries
11. Blueberries
12. Green beans

If you can't or will not buy organic produce, consider these food prep precautions:

*Scrub them in cold water. Rinse fruit and vegetables in cold water while scrubbing them with a soft brush can remove some pesticide residues.

*Baking soda. The results of a research study published in 2017 in the *Journal of Agricultural and Food Chemistry* showed that soaking apples in a baking soda solution (1 teaspoon of baking soda in 2 liters of water) for 12 to 15 minutes removed up to 96% of pesticide residues.

*Vinegar. Add one cup of white vinegar for each 3 cups of water. Let produce soak for 20 minutes. Rinse and wipe with a clean cloth or paper towel.

*Peel fruits and vegetables: For those fruits and vegetables where it's reasonable, taking off the skin can significantly reduce dietary intake of pesticide residues.

*Blanching produce (exposing it to boiling, then cold water) may significantly reduce pesticide residue levels in vegetables and fruit except peaches.

Buy organic produce, wild-caught fish, and grass-fed livestock meats with no hormones.

EWG.org's 2024 *Clean 15* list of non-organic fruits and vegetables with the least contamination of pesticides and herbicides:
1. Avocados
2. Sweet Corn
3. Pineapples
4. Frozen Sweet Peas
5. Onions
6. Papayas
7. Eggplants
8. Asparagus
9. Kiwis
10. Cabbage
11. Cauliflower
12. Mushrooms
13. Honeydew Melons
14. Cantaloupes
15. Broccoli

Warning! Heavy Metals Contamination

In his book *Food Forensics*, Mike Adams (also known as the "Health Ranger") highlights widespread contamination in American foods, identifying that a significant percentage of common foods contain harmful substances. Adams suggests that contamination, especially with heavy metals and toxic chemicals, is alarmingly prevalent, impacting more than 80% of certain food categories. His tests focus on heavy metals like lead, mercury, cadmium, and arsenic, particularly in processed and imported foods.

These are among the top foods he found to be the most contaminated:

1. Protein powders – Often contaminated with heavy metals like lead and cadmium.

2. Rice and rice-based products – High levels of arsenic, especially in products like rice protein.

3. Seafood (especially larger fish like tuna and swordfish) – Known for mercury contamination.

4. Chocolate and cocoa powder – Cadmium and lead contamination are common, particularly in imported brands.

5. Superfoods and green powders – Heavy metals like lead and arsenic contamination, especially in products from overseas.

6. Baby foods – Arsenic, cadmium, and lead levels have been found in rice-based baby foods and juices.

7. Imported fruits and vegetables – Pesticides and heavy metals are more likely in produce from countries with lax safety standards.

8. Herbal supplements – Some brands may contain heavy metals and other toxins, especially in products sourced from Asia.

9. Spices (like turmeric and cinnamon) – Lead and other contaminants are often found, especially in products that are adulterated or cheaply sourced.

10. Fruit juices (especially apple juice) – Arsenic contamination has been frequently reported, often from imported sources.

The findings in *Food Forensics* have fueled discussions about food safety, particularly concerning products from countries with less rigorous safety regulations. Adams calls for more transparency and stricter testing for food contaminants to better protect public health.

Superfoods for Your Consideration

I posted this as an internet search: "Top 10 most healthful foods - cite three agreeing sources for each." I looked for those foods that appeared unanimously --- or almost --- on every list. Additionally, I cross-referenced healthy food suggestions from my many listed healthcare and cancer experts. Though there are other super healthy foods, here is a list of "must" foods for your longevity game plan:

1. Berries, particularly blueberries. Also, strawberries and raspberries.

2. Legumes, particularly lentils and various varieties of beans.

3. Cruciferous vegetables, particularly broccoli, Brussels sprouts, and cauliflower.

4. Whole grains, particularly oats and quinoa. Beware of wheat because of herbicide and pesticide spray contamination and GMO (Genetically Modified Organisms) prevalence. Avoid GMO crops to be safe.

5. Nuts & Seeds, particularly almonds, walnuts, cashews, chia seeds, and ground flax seeds.

6. Wild salmon and other oily fish, like sardines and mackerel. Absolutely no farm-raised fish.

7. Leafy greens, particularly spinach and kale.

8. Avocadoes and extra virgin olive oil are both sources of healthy, necessary monosaturated fats.

9. Sweet potatoes

10. Organic whole milk plain yogurt or plain Greek yogurt with no sweeteners or emulsifiers.

Honorable Mention Super Foods in my research:

1. Eggs, hormone-free from free-range chickens

2. Organic apples

3. Tomatoes

4. Garlic

5. Green Tea

6. Dark chocolate

Budget for Healthy Foods

The three Big Lures in the modern Western diet are taste, convenience, and cost.

Busy, activity-filled lives and/or laziness draw many toward the convenience of prepared fast-food joints or processed foods that come in a box, bag, or can that we can heat in the microwave. And they taste sooooo good with the added sugars and sweeteners! I've been there, answering the siren's call, but I now fight these temptations. I suggest you do, too.

Also, the expense of dining on fast food, processed carbs, and sugar is usually less costly compared to healthy food purchases and their required prep time. However, this does not mean that any foods are cheap.

Interestingly, when the annual US inflation rate is officially announced each year by the US Bureau of Labor Statistics (BLS), the rates seem comically low. Here are the "official" inflation rates for recent years: 2021: 4.7%, 2022: 8%, 2023: 4.1%, 2024: projected to be around 2.4%. Hmmm.

Do you know the two categories of goods that are NOT included in the calculation of the annual US inflation rate? Things we use every day --- energy and food!!!!!!!! Our necessary daily commodities.

I read an article published on June 26, 2024, about a TikTok user posting as @sewerlidd. With the receipt in hand, the user posted a video comparing their Walmart grocery bill in 2022 to how much the same order would cost today in 2024. In 2022, the purchased items cost $126, but now it would cost $414, nearly four times the price of their original order, an inflation rate of a whopping 328% over 2 years! In other terms, according to the post, food prices at Walmart have more than tripled in two years.

In 2024, I rarely dine out. From my perspective, this experience has become insanely expensive, besides possibly unhealthy. Even if I order an entrée salad, I have no idea about the pesticides and herbicides on the lettuce and other condiment components. I would rather save my cash to buy organic, unsprayed foods, unwilling to put a price limit on my health and active longevity.

So, Health Warrior, save your money and your health by not buying poison "food" or, at least, consider reducing your dining out frequency and processed foods consumption.

Fasting for Health, Recovery, and Prevention

Fasting has vital cancer-fighting and recuperative benefits.

1. Enhanced Cellular Repair and Longevity

*Fasting triggers autophagy, a process where cells clean out damaged components, potentially reducing the risk of age-related diseases such as Alzheimer's, Parkinson's, and cancer.

*Intermittent fasting can potentially extend lifespan by improving metabolic and cellular health.

2. Improved Metabolic Health

*Fasting improves insulin sensitivity, helping regulate blood sugar levels and reducing the risk of type 2 diabetes.

*By reducing calorie intake and enhancing fat metabolism, fasting supports weight loss and helps maintain a healthy body composition.

3. Reduced Inflammation

*Fasting lowers inflammatory markers in the body, which may help prevent or alleviate chronic conditions like heart disease, arthritis, and inflammatory bowel disease.

4. Brain Health

*Fasting may promote the production of brain-derived neurotrophic factor (BDNF), a protein linked to improved brain function and resilience to neurodegenerative diseases.

*Improved focus and mental clarity during fasting are attributed to ketones, an alternative energy source for the brain when glucose levels drop.

5. Hormonal and Heart Health

*Fasting boosts levels of human growth hormone (HGH), which supports muscle growth, fat loss, and tissue repair

*Fasting can reduce risk factors like blood pressure, cholesterol, and triglyceride levels, improving cardiovascular health.

I suspect when most people hear of fasting, they associate this with food deprivation for a full day or days. Though refraining from consuming only clean distilled water for a day or more has great health benefits, it is more reasonable and less terrifying for most people --- be they healthy or healing --- to use a 16/8 fasting regimen in which you do all your eating entirely within an 8-hour window. For instance, choose an 8-hour span on the clock, like 9:30 am to 5:30 pm, in which you eat healthy foods in reasonable portions. Then, for 16 hours, you eat nothing but stay magnificently hydrated with clean water.

An additional benefit of finishing your eating hours before bedtime is that you will sleep better since your body is not busy with digestion.

SUMMARY OF "MUST-DOs" TO INCLUDE IN YOUR WRITTEN BATTLE PLAN

A cancer-fighting battle plan involves a comprehensive approach to prevention, early detection, treatment, and lifestyle changes. Here's a sample plan. Always consider vetting these suggestions with medical, nutritional, and health professionals. Continue your diligent research, reading, listening, watching, and learning. Expand the points below in your Battle Plan, and fill in the details. Don't limit your plan to only these "must-dos." These are only critical starting points:

1. Affirm your will and passionate reasons for living. Clarify, write, and read daily your Noble Purpose. Know why the world needs you and your gifts & talents.

2. Take charge of your health. YOU are the battlefield general. Your doctor is not God. He or she is your dutiful soldier ally. Effective, health-restoring cancer-treating alternatives are many and growing in number. Fight for your health!

3. Adopt a healthy diet. Focus on whole foods, including a variety of fruits, vegetables, whole grains, and lean proteins. Minimize processed foods, sugars, refined carbohydrates, and processed meats. Consider incorporating anti-inflammatory and antioxidant-rich foods like berries, leafy greens, cruciform vegetables, nuts, and seeds. Buy organic and/or grow your own food. Organics are more expensive, but how much is your health worth? Farming herbicides and pesticides on produce can prompt and encourage cancer. Wash fruits and vegetables in vinegar or baking powder solutions mentioned previously. Check out the "Dirty Dozen" and "Clean 15" at EWG.org.

4. Create a fasting window. The cancer-fighting benefits of fasting are proven. Start slowly, if necessary, by doing all of your eating within a 10-hour window during the day, making sure to finish several hours before bedtime. Stive to eventually restrict your eating to an 8-hour window. At all times, stay hydrated with clean water.

5. Vitamins and supplements. Even with a healthy diet, you may need insurance your body has healthy levels of vitamins, minerals, and nutrients. Among others, research and consider vitamins A, B, C, D, E, zinc, magnesium, CO-Q10, NAC (N-Acetyl-Cysteine), Quercetin, Selenium, Omega-3's, Resveratrol, Turmeric/Curcumin, and healthy-gut probiotics.

6. Stay adequately hydrated. A typical formula for daily water consumption: body weight in pounds / 2 = ounces of water to be consumed. Consider a countertop water distiller to remove impurities from your tap or well water. Make sure all components of the distiller that might contact the water, including the receptacle pitcher, are made of metal or glass, not plastic. Tip: Set the alarm on your cell phone to sound hourly as a reminder to drink water.

7. Exercise regularly. Aim for at least 150 minutes of moderate-intensity exercise or 75 minutes of vigorous exercise weekly. Activities like walking, swimming, or cycling can reduce cancer risk. Set the alarm on your cell phone to sound hourly as a reminder to get up and move. If you have a pet dog, daily outdoor walks will necessarily be part of your dog's care. And there may be added health-enhancing social interactions when people inquire about and dote on your beloved pet. Tip: Set the alarm on your cell phone to sound hourly as a reminder to get up and move.

8. Maintain a healthy weight. Obesity is a known risk factor for several types of cancer. Regular physical activity combined with a balanced diet helps maintain a healthy weight. Check your bathroom scales frequently. Strive for a Body Mass Index (BMI) of less than 25.

9. Avoid tobacco, smoking marijuana, and vaping, and limit alcohol. Smoking is the leading cause of preventable cancer. Avoiding tobacco in all forms is crucial. Limit alcohol intake, as it is linked to an increased risk of several cancers.

10. Discover and avoid environmental toxins, including the air in your home. Limit exposure to known carcinogens such as asbestos, radon, airborne mold, and certain chemicals in household products. Take steps to eliminate toxins and opt for natural or organic products where possible, including using only fluoride-free toothpaste.

Do this: As often and as long as possible, open your home's windows and screened doors to flush the toxins out of your house or apartment, allowing for fresh air to circulate throughout.

11. Go outside often and experience Nature. Consider *grounding*, the practice of walking barefoot on grass, soil, rock, or the beach with nothing manmade between you and the natural ground.

12. Protect your skin. Low-angle, early morning and late evening sunshine is health-enhancing. However, intense UV radiation from the mid-day sun can be damaging. Melanoma and skin cancers can be virulent and deadly. Use sunscreen with an SPF of 30 or higher, wear protective clothing, and avoid tanning beds. Regularly check your skin for changes or new growths. Remember to protect the backs of your hands.

This being suggested, discover and use only sunscreens without harmful, sometimes carcinogenic, ingredients. Do your research.

13. Get regular physical health screenings. Follow recommended guidelines for cancer screenings like mammograms, colonoscopies, and Pap smears. Early detection increases the chances of successful treatment. Consider the Galleri Test, which screens for 50 different cancers to reveal them long before symptoms might appear.

14. Mental health maintenance. At least two studies indicate that up to 25% of cancer patients are afflicted with depression, preventing them from effectively helping themselves. This number naturally increases as physical pain and fear accelerate. If you are a cancer patient's advocate, you will be necessarily involved in getting help for your friend or loved one.

15. Manage stress. Chronic stress can weaken the immune system. Incorporate stress-reducing practices like meditation, deep breathing, yoga, or hobbies you enjoy.

*Caring for and interacting with your beloved pet is a proven stress reliever.

16. Practice gratitude. Even though you have challenges, recount your blessings, which may include family, friends, beloved pets, education, intelligence, opportunities, financial stability, your home, Nature, sunshine, and the overlooked little things, such as sight, hearing, and taste.

17. Socialize often with friends and family. Join a club or Meetup group. Volunteer. Actively giving and receiving loving interactions boosts immunity and adds meaning and purpose to our lives.

18. Keep your brain and cognitive function sharp. Your brain needs daily exercise. Challenge yourself mentally and learn something new every day. Read, write, or enjoy word or number games like Sudoku, Wordscapes, crossword puzzles, Strands, Spelling Bee, or card games involving numbers.

19. Boost your immune function. Focus on a nutrient-rich diet, regular exercise, adequate & quality sleep, and vitamins & supplements, like vitamins C and D, zinc picolinate, elderberry, and gut-health probiotics.

*Staying on the move and exercising is imperative.

*Loving human interactions and stress relief definitely boosts immune health.

*Studies have demonstrated that the loving interaction between you and your pet boosts your immune system.

*Quality sleep is a necessary component of excellent immune function.

20. Quality sleep is imperative. 7 – 9 hours of quality sleep is crucial for improving quality of life, managing cancer symptoms and side effects, boosting your immune system, and enhancing your treatment response. Sleep disruption is common in cancer patients due to stress, anxiety, and treatment side effects. Address sleep issues by establishing a consistent sleep schedule and seeking medical advice if excessive sleepiness or insomnia persists. Reduce time spent on TV, computer, and cellphone screens before bed. Good sleep practices are vital in your individualized cancer battle plan.

Personally, I sleep happy and sweetly with my precious Squeaky Cat snuggled against my torso, purring through the night.

21. Oral health maintenance. Do not underestimate the importance of a healthy mouth for assisting the immune system, curbing the spread of infections transferred to the circulatory system, maintaining a healthy gut environment, and disease prevention. Floss thoroughly and brush every day. Avoid fluoride toothpastes. Get regular dental check-ups that check for infections and gum disease.

22. Keep your gut health and microbiome bulletproof. The microbiome refers to the collection of microorganisms bacteria, viruses, fungi, and other microbes --- that live on and inside the human body, including the mouth and the gut. According to Harvard Health, unhealthy disruptions and imbalances in the gut's microbiome are associated with conditions such as inflammatory bowel disease (IBD), obesity, diabetes, allergies, and even cancer. Microbiome-based therapies, like probiotics, prebiotics, and maintaining good oral health, can aid the immune system to fight and heal disease.

23. Stay informed and advocate for your health. Research is a never-ending endeavor. Educate yourself about the latest research on cancer prevention and treatments. Know what is possible. Communicate openly with your healthcare provider, and don't hesitate to seek second opinions or explore integrative therapies.

24. Do the necessary hard work every day driven by your Noble Purpose. Laziness and everyday distractions will seek to derail you. Be alert and determined.

25. Refuse to be ordinary!

This plan does NOT exclude professional medical advice but can serve as a foundation for your Master Battle Plan for healing, reducing cancer risk, and supporting optimal health.

Fight on, my warrior brothers and sisters! The world needs you, your passions, your gifts, and your inspirational winning example.

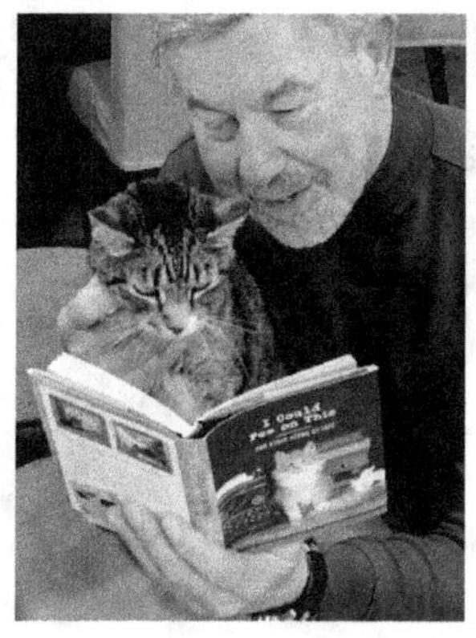

MichaelGormanBooks.com

*History: **Unexpected Detours and Interesting Connections in Today's History Highlights**, a series

*Health: **I Said "Hell No!" to the Grim Reaper: 200 Hacks for Your Optimal Health and Living Beyond 100 Years**
   99 Simple, At-Home Health Hacks to Help You Live Actively Beyond 100 Years
   Optimal Health and Longevity: Adopting Battle Tactics from Sun Tsu's The Art of War, vol. 1

Growth & Betterment: **Noble Life Purpose: Discover It, Live It for a Happy Life**
   How to Be Happy Alone But Not Lonely
   Emotional Healing: My Story, My Solution
   Getting Over the Breakup & Finding Happiness
   Loneliness --- Kick the Hell Out of It

Fly Fishing: **Steelhead Fly Angling, Guerilla Tactics**
   Effective Stilwater Fly Fishing, An Analytical Approach
   American Nymph Fly-Fishing Guide

One final time. Turn the page →

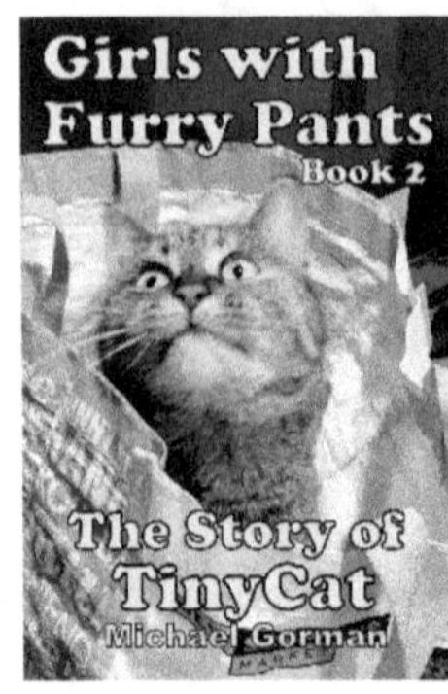

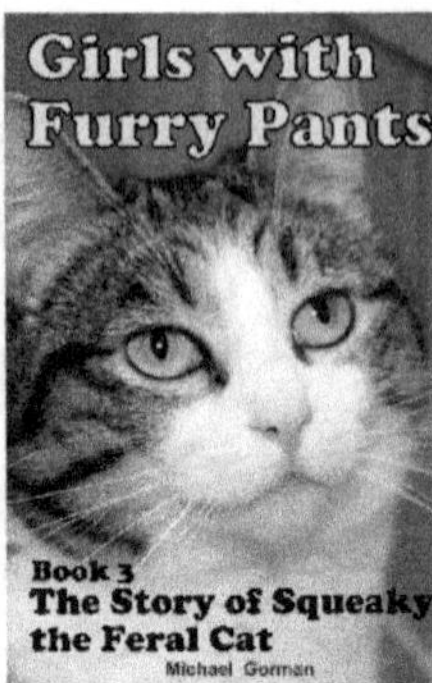

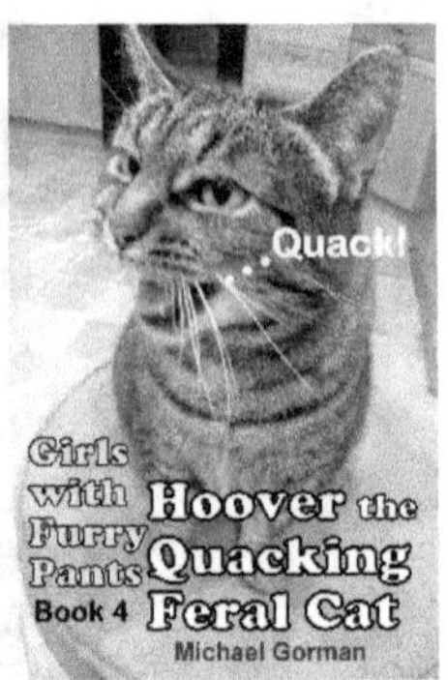

MICHAEL GORMAN CAT BOOKS
AVAILABLE AT MICHAELGORMANBOOKS.COM
OR AMAZON

Taming Feral Cats – 10 Easy Steps

Taming Feral Cats – My Loving Plan for Squeaky

Taming Feral Cats – My Loving Plan for Hoover the Quacking Feral Cat

Don't Eat My Cat! The Story of Bub, the Wonder Boy

The Girls with Furry Pants series ---

Book 1 – The Story of Miracle Cat

Book 2 – The Story of TinyCat

Book 3 – The Story of Squeaky the Feral Cat

Book 4 – Hoover the Quacking Feral Cat

MichaelGormanBooks.com

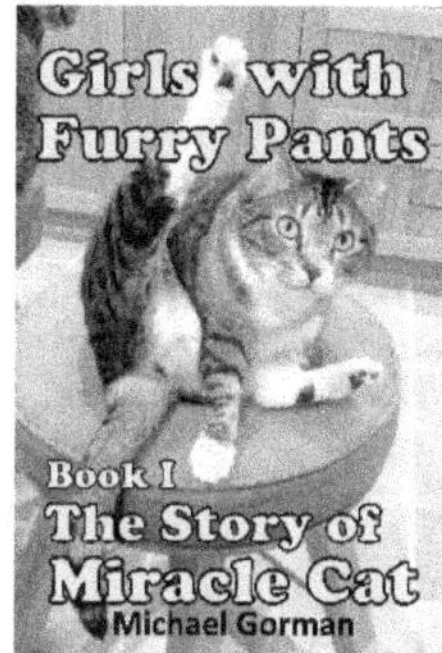
Girls with
Furry Pants
Book I
The Story of
Miracle Cat
Michael Gorman

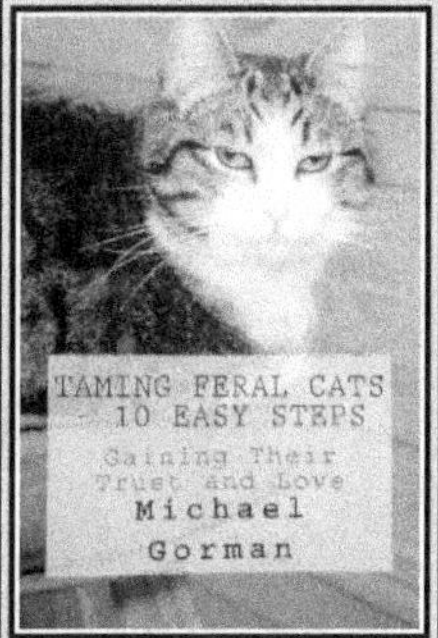
TAMING FERAL CATS
10 EASY STEPS
Gaining Their
Trust and Love
Michael
Gorman

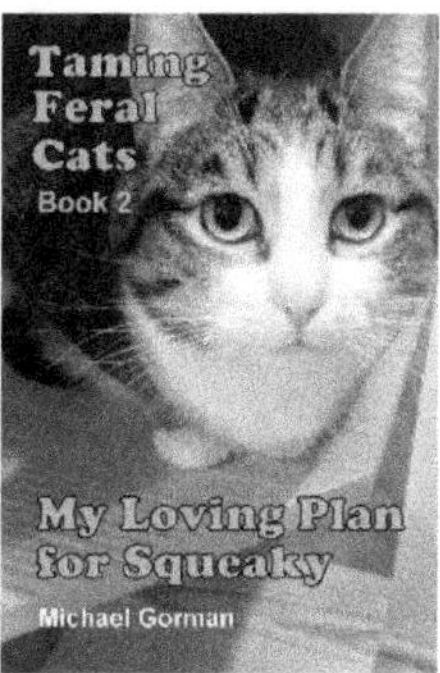
Taming
Feral
Cats
Book 2
My Loving Plan
for Squeaky
Michael Gorman

```
      (\___/)
   =(='.'=)=
   (")___(")
```

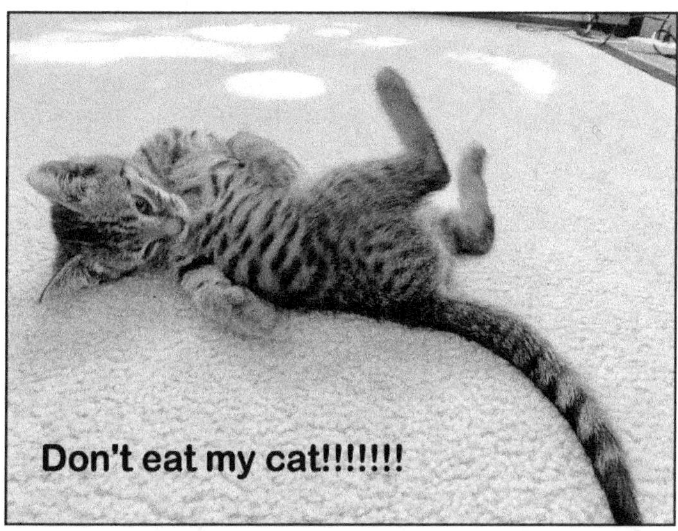
Don't eat my cat!!!!!!!!

Michael F Gorman

Cancer – YOU Must Be the Battlefield General